Praise for the BluePrintCleanse®

"BPC is a manageable, enjoyable, yummy-tasting cleanse. It's not torture like other fasts or cleanses; it gives me energy. And when I'm done, I don't crave a cheeseburger or pizza—I honestly crave healthier foods!"
—Christine Taylor, actress

"I love BPC more than wrapping myself in Saran Wrap and sleeping in a sauna!"
—Robert Verdi, celebrity stylist and television personality

"BluePrint is a user-friendly, regimented, efficient, healthy way to get back on track and improve the way you feel after you've done a little too much indulging. They couldn't make it easier for you!"
—Jim Gold, president/CEO, Bergdorf Goodman

"After a few decades of treating my body like a trash can, Blue-PrintCleanse was just what I needed to kick-start a sane, healthy, restorative year. The BluePrintCleanse has become a trusted tool in my continued effort to reclaim my body and redefine my complicated relationship with food."
—Edward Ugel, author of *I'm with Fatty: Losing Fifty Pounds in Fifty Miserable Weeks*

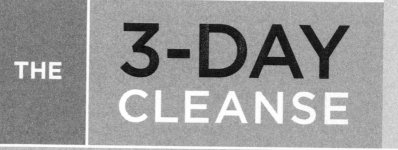

THE 3-DAY CLEANSE

DRINK FRESH JUICE,
EAT REAL FOOD, AND GET BACK
INTO YOUR SKINNY JEANS

ZOË SAKOUTIS
& ERICA HUSS

WELLNESS CENTRAL

New York Boston

Neither this cleanse nor any other cleansing program should be followed without first consulting a health care professional. If you have any special conditions requiring attention, you should consult with your health care professional regularly regarding possible modification of the program contained in this book.

Wellness Central
Hachette Book Group
237 Park Avenue
New York, NY 10017

www.HachetteBookGroup.com

Wellness Central is an imprint of Grand Central Publishing.
The Wellness Central name and logo are trademarks of Hachette Book Group, Inc.

Printed in the United States of America

First Edition: March 2010
10 9 8 7 6 5 4 3 2 1

Library of Congress Cataloging-in-Publication Data

Sakoutis, Zoë.
   The 3-day cleanse : drink fresh juice, eat real food, and get back into your skinny jeans / Zoë Sakoutis and Erica Huss.—1st ed.
      p. cm.
   ISBN 978-0-446-54571-6
   1. Detoxification (Health)   2. Fruit juices.   3. Vegetable juices.   I. Huss, Erica.   II. Title.
   RA784.5.S25 2010
   613.2—dc22
                                                     2009021967

"You must have discipline to have fun."
—Julia Child

Love, Zoë and Erica

Contents

Acknowledgments

Special thanks to Team BPC: Elvin Acosta, Ricardo Alvarez, Damon Alves, Carlos Aparicilo, Patrick Burlingham, Stephanie Campione, Andres Campos, Anthony Costa, Emily Eddins, Waleed Gettes, Andres Gonzales, Erin Greenman, Balaram Hariyogam, Christian Henderson, David Hodorowski, Alexandra Holmes, Keith Irwin, Jose Lema, Manuel Lema, Fernando Lopez, Sarah Main, Brian Martinez, Sunilda Rodriguez, Jesus Rojas, Juan Rojas, Jose Roldan, Victoria Salemo, Maggie Schanck

Bartenders throughout lower Manhattan and Brooklyn for making the writing process that much more inspiring
CI for all of your love and support!
Lisa, Jolise, Ian, and Douglas Sakoutis
Linda Jo + Big Mike, for always letting me hang from the monkey bars with no hands
Kristen Reyes
Rebecca Isenberg
Shira, Princess of Power
Mark Wood, the Magic Caterpillar
The Waverly
The Maritime

Schrager

S/'wichcraft

Kern + Lead

Zipcar

Joe the Juice Bottle Man

Chris Stasinos wherever you are... we will find you.

Louisa S.

Natalie Kaire

DJ Debra, aka Spinderella

Kung Fu Panda

Karaoke

McDonald's, Burger King, Taco Bell, KFC, Pfizer, the FDA, and yellow dye 2 for making what we do that much more necessary

Introduction

ZOË: In 2000, I greeted the new millennium not with a popping cork but with a nasty cold. It was just the latest in a long string of annoying illnesses, aches, and pains. A sore back. A chronic cough. Frequent headaches. Fatigue.

A friend of mine who was a devout raw foodist suggested I do a seven-day juice cleanse/fast to rid my body of the toxins that were making me sick. I was skeptical, but decided I had nothing to lose (except a week of food and, possibly, a few pounds), so I tried it. Although the end results of the cleanse were fantastic, I found the process itself to be excruciatingly painful. As my body detoxed, all the poisons came to the surface. I had terrible migraines and felt bloated, and my skin was breaking out. My cold got worse because everything was trying to exit my body very quickly—all at once! Later, I tried the Master Cleanse, which is primarily water with lemon and maple syrup. This wasn't quite as bad because I'd prepared, but about four days in, a fungus appeared on my cheek. This was no doubt due to the fact that I was flooding my body with maple syrup—essentially cooked sugar, a favorite food for fungi.

I realized that the reason I suffered such effects during the cleanse was that the process itself was simply too extreme.

At the time, I was *not* a vegan or a raw foodist; I wasn't even a vegetarian! I worked hard and played hard, eating whatever I wanted whenever I wanted. I was in college and New York City was my campus—my habits didn't exactly include yoga and salads. I worked as a bartender throughout college, mixing the opposite of green juice. I went out a lot, I partied with friends, I stayed up all night writing papers. I knew my body needed help.

The question was: How could I get the benefits of the cleansing without undergoing the agony I experienced during these cleanses? Because, to be totally honest, given how awful I felt that week, I was really hesitant to try it again.

And yet I realized that to be truly effective, a cleanse had to be more than just a one-time painful experience that you never wanted to repeat. It also couldn't be so extreme that it totally dictated your life, kept you in your house for the duration, and led your friends to avoid you for fear you'd bite their heads off.

Cleansing and how good I felt afterward had another benefit: It made me realize the benefits of nutrition. So I went back to school and became a certified nutritional consultant, changed my eating habits, embraced raw foodism and, eventually, food combining (more on that later). But I never got the idea of cleansing out of my head.

The more I thought about it, the more I realized that I (and most of the people I knew) needed a cleansing option that was easy, tasted good, felt good, and made me want to do it again and again. It also needed to provide enough nutritional sustenance so I could continue my normal life—friends, work, exercise.

ERICA: Zoë was talking about this with everyone she knew, including me. We had been friends for more than seven years. A fellow foodie, I was on my own career path in public relations for chefs, restaurants, and wine brands. Our skill sets were a natural fit, and together we rolled up our sleeves, did a test run with our friends and families, and created what is known as the BluePrintCleanse.

*   *   *

The BluePrintCleanse was the first line of juice cleanses in the country to offer varying levels of intensity depending on an individual's dietary habits and history. It's a user-friendly system of cleansing designed to be practical for all nutritional lifestyles, from the most austere of raw food acolytes to the burger-and-red-wine crowd that needs to occasionally offset the damage from their indulgences.

Today our Manhattan-based juice detox delivery service is used by thousands of clients throughout the metropolitan area and the country. It's been written up in nearly every major media outlet, including *Domino, People, Allure, Cosmopolitan, Fit Yoga, Conde Nast Traveler, Vogue,* and *New York* magazines. It has been featured on *Good Morning America, NBC New York,* and *ABC News.* Why? Because it is so easy, so commonsense, and so beneficial.

Our clients have their fresh-squeezed juices delivered right to their door with just a couple of days' notice. They find that whether they do a 3-Day, 5-Day, or 10-Day Cleanse, whether they choose the easiest Level 1 or the most advanced Level 3, at the end they have more energy, clearer skin, a more focused mind, and feel completely amazing.

Our clients rave about our Cleanse, most encourage their friends to try it, and nearly all return to do it again and again.

But we know that not everyone can afford our juices as often as they would like. We also can't send them *everywhere* there are people who'd like to try them. That's why we wrote *The 3-Day Cleanse,* so that you, too, will be able to reap all the BluePrint-Cleanse benefits by following our renowned program in your own home.

This book not only details the reasons *why* you should cleanse, what the expected benefits will be, and what medical science says about cleansing and fasting, but provides a detailed, step-by-step regimen for before, during, and after the Cleanse.

We have more than a hundred recipes in this book for everything from the juices needed for the Cleanse itself to salads, entrées, and side dishes to help you prepare for and come out of the Cleanse. These recipes will allow you to enjoy your own customized Cleanse, tailor-made to your personal health and time frame. The ingredients are easy to find and the recipes are simple. And the juices are so good that your friends will actually be clamoring for a taste.

Of course, these are all incredibly healthy foods we hope you'll consume between cleansings, because *The 3-Day Cleanse* is not *just* about the Cleanse itself. It's also about making easy lifestyle changes that will make you healthier and feel better. For example, in the final chapter, we introduce you to the food combining philosophy, a way of eating that has, at its core, the understanding that certain foods should be eaten separately so as to enhance overall digestion. This is an important part of our philosophy that we can promise will yield effective results—even when you're not cleansing.

We're pretty sure that by the time you finish the book and your first Cleanse, you, too, will come over to our philosophy: Work hard. Play hard. Cleanse. Repeat.

—Zoë Sakoutis and Erica Huss

THE PROGRAM

CHAPTER 1

It's a Dirty World Out There (and In There)

The increased clarity was gradual, from day to day, so I didn't really notice the change as acutely as I did as soon as I began to eat solid food again. That was like getting knocked off a tall fence; I literally felt my consciousness drop a few notches. Nevertheless, now being completely devoid of toxins, I was leagues ahead of my peer group. I know I can use this knowledge of cleansing whenever I need a higher level of awareness. This program is so much more than merely a weight-loss or a detox tool. It is really a way to get to your higher consciousness in the same way meditation does, but the effort is easier and the effect lasts much longer.

—SHARON, A BLUEPRINTCLEANSE CLIENT

We know you're excited to dive right into the "how" of *The 3-Day Cleanse*. And we're excited to show you what you need to do to get started. But before we go there, it's important that you understand a bit more about *why* cleansing is so important. That's the focus of this chapter. You'll learn exactly how ubiquitous and prevalent toxins are (you can't get away from them even if you're vegan and eat only organic). You'll also learn (with a minimum of the "ick" factor) just how your digestive system works, so you can better understand how important regular Cleanses are in maintaining the health of that system.

Let's start with the food supply.

When was the last time you ate something you could identify with one word? Something whose ingredients list was either nonexistent or less than four items, all of which you could pronounce? Something that actually looked like a food that your ancestors might have eaten a thousand or more years ago?

The truth is that today's food supply is sadly out of sync with our bodies' nutritional needs. Loaded with salt and sugar (did you know that there is more salt in breakfast cereal than in some brands of potato chips?), filled with chemicals designed to preserve and plump, dehydrated, modified, enhanced...the food most Americans put into their bodies affords as many health benefits as drinking a bottle of sewer sludge.

Can you imagine, then, what that sludge does to the inner workings of your body, from your digestive system to your respiratory system to the brain itself?

No wonder rates of obesity and diabetes are off the charts and allergies and autoimmune diseases are on the rise. No surprise that conditions such as irritable bowel syndrome, fibromyalgia, chronic fatigue syndrome, and other ailments—some of which didn't even exist fifty years ago—affect millions of people today. No, we're not suggesting that the food itself causes these diseases (except, maybe, in the case of obesity), but that the type of food we keep shoveling into our mouths is so toxic, so far from the "natural" ingredients our bodies were designed to digest, that we have created a toxic environment within ourselves, one that affects every aspect of our ability to stave off disease even as it ages us faster.

The toxins accumulating in our bodies are not limited to those found on grocery store shelves, however. They also come from the water we drink, the air we breathe, and the way we live.

So listen up, ladies and gentlemen. It's time to sweep away the dirt and open up the view. Time to clear out the crap and restore your body to its peak operating ability.

It's time to cleanse and restore.

The benefit? An improved ability to fight off disease, reduce inflammation, and slow aging. Once you learn to regularly clear out your body with the Cleanse, we promise you this: You will look better, you will feel better, and you will understand the difference between feeling full and feeling *nourished*. You'll weigh less, brim with more energy, and look and feel sexier!

Welcome to the new you.

I went on the Cleanse because I had a terrible allergic reaction to some medication my doctor prescribed. After getting treatment for that, three days later I contracted a massive intestinal virus due to the original medication I took to combat the initial ailment! I was

rushed to the emergency room suffering from severe dehydration.
I decided not to fill the antibiotics prescribed (the last thing I
wanted was more medication) and, after a week of recovering, did
my first 3-day BluePrintCleanse.

After the Cleanse, I felt healthier than even before that horrible
allergic reaction. I am no longer bloated, my skin is clear, and I
have plenty of energy. I am definitely making the BluePrintCleanse
a regular practice in my health regime. Just as great is the fact that
I'm also back in my "skinny" jeans!

—SHARI, A BLUEPRINTCLEANSE CLIENT

CLEANSING WHAT?

Before we get more into the whys and wherefores of the Cleanse
and cleansing itself, let's talk a bit about just what it is—and
what it's not.

The BluePrintCleanse is a very simple, yet effective program built around fruit and vegetable juices. Although we sell
freshly prepared juices to clients around the country, we've
designed the program in this book so you can get all the benefits
of the BluePrintCleanse at home. All you need is a juicer, this
book, organic produce, and a few minutes a day to whip up the
juices.

Then, after preparing, you spend anywhere from one to ten
days or longer drinking nothing but fresh juice, water, and tea.
The juices you drink depend on which level of the Cleanse you
choose. So whether this is your first or your fourteenth Cleanse,
there is a level that's right for you.

When you finish the Cleanse, you gradually reintroduce solid
food to your body for a few days before resuming your normal
eating habits.

As you'll see throughout the book, however, the 3-Day Cleanse
is *not* a one-time thing, but a way of living, a lifestyle, something

you should integrate into your life just as you integrate exercise. The promise of the 3-Day Cleanse is that it will change forever how you think about your body and food.

An important distinction here: The Cleanse is *not* a fast. Maybe you've heard of other "fasts" or cleanses out there that are composed primarily of lemon juice, cayenne pepper, and maple syrup. In our opinion, these fasts are much too extreme. They lead to uncomfortable, sometimes harmful, detoxification side effects such as fatigue, skin eruptions, and migraines. The simple fact is that not everyone can handle these "extreme" cleanses. They are just too much for most people who are used to the typical American diet, which includes meat and dairy (as well as alcohol and lots of sugar). Maybe if you're already following a vegetarian, vegan, and/or raw food diet, you can tolerate this type of fast, but even then, you will find the process somewhat challenging.

It's important for your readers to know that I tried two water-based "fasts" before and the experiences were awful. Both times I spent a day or two in bed, throwing up, with diarrhea. The authors who recommended this regime assured their readers that it was just the toxins leaving their bodies and we shouldn't be concerned. Perhaps that's true, but I don't believe it's healthy for the human body to experience such severe symptoms unless there is a serious health crisis to deal with. Juicing alleviates this kind of misery.

—RACHEL

The 3-Day Cleanse is *not* about self-denial. We both have a great appreciation for the pleasures of good food. That's why our juices and the recipes we provide are, dare we say, *delicious*. Just ask anyone! The fruit juices are sweet yet have no added sugar, the vegetable juices taste so fresh you'd swear you were eating veggies in the middle of a farmer's market, and our nut milks have been compared to ice cream and other desserts— *that's* how good they are!

The 3-Day Cleanse is *not* a weight-loss program (although you *will* lose weight if you have it to lose). We hate to tell you this, but we didn't count calories when we developed the three levels of Cleanses. Nor did we count carbs or fat grams. We just developed our juices using the freshest ingredients available with the biggest detox bang-for-the-buck. Of course, you may lose a few pounds while on the Cleanse (more on that in Chapter 2). And it so happens that a lean body tends to be a healthier body. Plus, of course, the more of your diet that is derived from Mother Nature, the more likely you are to reach and maintain a healthy weight.

Finally, as we already said, the 3-Day Cleanse is *not* a one-time thing. Instead, the Cleanse is a new way of thinking about your body, your lifestyle, and your diet. One that recognizes the temptations that fill our world, the weaknesses in our current nutritional system, and the stresses upon our bodies. One that offers up simple, easy-to-use options to fight back against those seemingly intractable forces.

You'll read much more about the Cleanse itself and other life-changing habits the Cleanse can bring you in later chapters, including how to choose the cleansing program that's best for you, how to prepare for it, and how to do it. What we want to do here is reassure you that the programs we offer will be ones you can maintain throughout your life without having to compromise your lifestyle. The biggest change you'll find will be within yourself as you wake up to the possibility of living and functioning without the toxic sludge you've been unknowingly hauling around for years.

> ## "Is the Cleanse for Me?"
>
> The Cleanse is for everyone *except* people taking blood thinners, because the greens in our juice contain large amounts of vitamin K, which can interfere with anti-clotting medications. Also, people with diabetes should not do the Cleanse alone because of the amount of carbohydrates contained in the juice. Check with your doctor, however; you may be able to supplement your diet with the juices. Also, women who are pregnant or breastfeeding should not attempt the Cleanse as their only nutrition; you need more calories than it provides. And finally, children should not do an exclusive Cleanse because of the variety of foods they need for adequate growth, although they may also supplement with the juices.

IT'S A TOXIC WORLD

What is a toxin?

A toxin is a poisonous substance that is harmful to your body. There are man-made toxins such as pesticides and gasoline, and natural toxins such as those that result from the activities of daily living. There are also toxins in the food you eat and the water you drink (think chlorine, lead, and even the remnants of pharmaceutical medications!).

If you don't get rid of toxins in your body, they build up and damage cells and tissue, leading to diseases such as cancer, Alzheimer's disease, and heart disease. That's why your body has developed over time its own natural detoxification system composed of the liver, kidneys, intestines, and skin and described later in the chapter. Until about a hundred years ago, it worked pretty well. That's because we ate what we grew and raised (with no excess chemicals, hormones, or drugs added), our air and water were cleaner, and our lives were calmer.

Today, however, our built-in detox system can easily become overwhelmed by the thousands of toxins it is exposed to on a daily basis. The result? Illness, fatigue, headaches, mood disorders, and those nagging pains that let you know that something *just isn't right*.

Toxins make you sick through their effects at the cellular level. Two of the main avenues through which they wreak their damage are oxidative stress and inflammation.

Oxidative Stress

The best way to think about oxidative stress is to picture what happened to that shovel you left out in the garden all winter. Come spring, the once-bright metal was dull with rust. That rust occurred as oxygen molecules in the air interacted with the molecules in the metal, damaging the iron molecules and resulting in rust.

The same kind of thing happens in your body. As cells make energy, clear out toxins, fight off invaders, etc., they create their own toxic by-products called free radicals. Think of them as the exhaust emanating from cellular engines. These free radicals are highly toxic. As they ping around, they seek to snatch electrons from healthy molecules so they can make themselves "whole" again. If they succeed, they damage those healthy molecules, in the process damaging the cell by attacking proteins, the DNA and nucleus of the cell, and the cell's membrane. This type of damage underlies conditions such as cancer, diabetes, Alzheimer's disease, and other chronic illnesses. It is called oxidative stress, a great name since it accurately describes what happens to those poor cells being nattered at by free radicals.

Luckily, your body has its own built-in protection system against oxidative stress: antioxidants. These scavenger molecules come from within your body and from the food you eat. You know them as vitamins A, C, and E; coenzyme Q-10; manganese; iodide; and plant-based chemicals called polyphenols. Their job is to scoop up free radicals and render them harmless.

This is why a balanced diet is so important to your health—without it, your body can't produce enough antioxidants to fight off oxidation. Not only that, but an *unhealthy* diet produces its own load of free radicals!

Here's where the 3-Day Cleanse comes in. Because the Cleanse is made with only fruits, vegetables, nuts, and other components high in antioxidants, with every Cleanse you get what amounts to a surge of antioxidants. These, in turn, provide extra protection against the oxidative stress that occurs as your body uses the Cleanse to flush away toxins from every nook and cranny.

There's an added bonus, too. Because the juices you consume on the Cleanse are so much easier to digest than your regular diet, less cellular energy is required for digestion and free radical production from digestion drops.

Inflammation

The second way toxins damage cells is through inflammation. The best way to describe inflammation is to think about what happens when you cut your finger. It bleeds for a bit and then becomes slightly red and warm to the touch. This is inflammation at work, a process your immune system uses to ward off bacteria, viruses, and other pathogens that could harm you and to repair cellular damage. Inflammation works great in the short term to fight infection; but it's not so great when it becomes chronic. Then it leads to such cellular overload and tissue damage that it contributes to conditions as diverse as heart disease, chronic pain, arthritis, and many brain-related conditions such as Parkinson's and Alzheimer's disease.

Any kind of toxin, whether internal or external, can jumpstart the inflammatory process and, once begun, make it go on longer than it should. Not only that, but the toxins themselves can make your immune system's response more intense than it should be.

This, in turn, can trigger autoimmunity, in which the immune system—which is only supposed to attack foreign compounds—begins attacking the body's own tissue. This is the process at work in diseases such as lupus, multiple sclerosis, and scleroderma. We think this may be one reason for the dramatic increase we've seen in autoimmune diseases, all of which have underlying inflammation as one of their hallmarks.

Unfortunately, inflammation and oxidation are not two separate processes but are inextricably linked. Inflammation leads to greater free radical production while oxidation triggers inflammation when the immune system rushes in to fix cells damaged through the oxidative process.

You don't want to suppress either system entirely; both have some positive benefits in your body or they wouldn't exist in the first place. The key with everything in your body—indeed, with everything in life—is moderation! The Cleanse gives each system a rest and helps strengthen your overall system to resist their negative effects.

Now let's take a closer look at some of those toxins.

Internal Detox

The feces that result at the end of digestion are one of your body's main ways of getting rid of toxins. The other three are urine, sweat, and breath. All depend on the main detoxification organs: the intestines, the liver, the kidneys, and the skin. We delve deeply into the role of the intestines beginning on page 32 when we discuss digestion. Now let's take a look at the other three.

THE LIVER

While the kidneys play an important role in detoxification, the star of your internal detox system is definitely the liver. In digestion it produces bile to break down fats. But the liver also breaks down and detoxifies drugs and alcohol as well as other toxins. That's why too many acetaminophen (Tylenol), too many cosmos, even exposure to the fumes of too many cleaning supplies can cause liver damage; you've simply exceeded its ability to filter out the bad stuff.

The liver uses various enzymes to break down toxins. The debris is then transported via bile to the intestines for removal. A word about liver enzymes: If you can't tolerate alcohol, or have severe sensitivities to perfumes, caffeine, or other chemicals, you may have low levels or low activity levels of liver enzymes. That's why it's important to enhance their activity through detoxification with the Cleanse. As you'll see in Chapter 3, our Cleanse juices are stocked with the nutrients essential for ensuring that liver enzymes work properly.

The amazing thing about the liver, however, is that because it is so important, it is the only organ able to regenerate, or re-create, itself. That's why people can donate a portion of their liver to someone for a liver transplant; their own liver will grow back like their hair or fingernails.

The liver is also quite amenable to its own detoxification. In fact, researchers are beginning to understand the science behind the use of herbs like milk thistle for "liver support." We'll talk more about these supportive herbs in Chapter 2.

THE KIDNEYS

Your kidneys have numerous roles to play in your body, not the least of which is maintaining the right fluid levels. This influences everything from blood pressure to nearly every physiologic process of daily life. The kidneys also act as a kind of Brita water purifier for the blood, removing excess water, salts, bile pigments, and cellular wastes for excretion as urine. That's why getting enough liquid, particularly water, is so important. Water serves as the transportation system to carry out toxins. The more water you consume, whether in food or drink, the more you pee and poop and the more toxins leave your body. Aim for at least six glasses a day, more when you're doing the Cleanse, exercising, or during warm weather. We'll talk more about water consumption during the Cleanse later.

THE SKIN

The skin is your largest organ, acting as a mini-excretory system by getting rid of urea (the waste product after protein metabolism), salts, and water through sweat. That's why exercise and sauna (described on page 26) are such excellent detoxification options.

The 3-Day Cleanse is designed to give all these detox organs a rest—in a very simple, delicious way!

THE MODERN FOOD SUPPLY

Over the past couple of years, we have found the hysteria related to the contamination of spinach with *E. coli* and tomatoes and peanut products with salmonella quite ironic. Ironic because these contaminants are all natural bugs that infest the food when regular sanitary conditions break down, yet we never see the same level of hysteria when, on a daily basis, our food supply is deliberately contaminated with pesticides, hormones, antibiotics, manufactured additives, and other such substances.

How toxic is our food supply? Well, in 2002 an environmental group estimated that about 20 percent of the entire U.S. food supply was contaminated with pesticide residue toxins, exposing the average American to these substances an average of sixty-eight times a day. Even organic foods are not exempt, with about 60 percent of sampled organic vegetables containing pesticide residue, although at much lower levels than commercially grown vegetables.

The fact is, thirty-seven of the pesticides approved for use on food supplies are neurotoxic, meaning they interfere with the activity of nerve cells like those found in the brain as well as throughout your body. Studies of animals and humans find exposure to these chemicals can lead to numerous behavioral and growth problems in children as well as cancer, reproductive changes, and memory and other cognitive problems in children and adults.

For instance, there's some evidence linking pesticides with breast and prostate cancers as well as soft-tissue tumors such as sarcoma, Hodgkin's lymphoma, and non-Hodgkin's lymphoma.

Pesticides fall in the category of POPs, persistent organic pollutants. That means they remain in the environment for years, decades, even centuries. Health effects now linked to POPs exposure include cancer, learning disorders, chronic health conditions, impaired immune function, reproductive dysfunction (i.e., low sperm counts and infertility), endometriosis, and diabetes. But pesticides can also lead to headaches, nausea, and simply "fuzzy thinking." It's why so many people say they simply "feel better" when they eat organic-only.

Pesticides aren't the only toxins you need to worry about, however. Food additives such as monosodium glutamate, dyes, and preservatives, while ostensibly safe, still put increased pressure on your detox system and may actually have serious health consequences.

The nonprofit Center for Science in the Public Interest (CSPI) published a list of the ten worst food additives in 1991. That list is still quite relevant today (and is updated regularly on the CSPI site at www.cspi.org). It includes acesulfame-K, sold under the brand name "Sunette" or "Sweet One" and found in baked goods, gum, gelatin desserts, and soft drinks and often used with another artificial sweetener, sucralose.

Consumer advocates were never satisfied with the kind of safety testing performed on acesulfame-K, some of which suggested the sweetener might cause cancer or affect the thyroid. But the Food and Drug Administration (FDA) approved its use in food products anyway.

Other items on the CSPI's list are the synthetic dyes used to color food. While one of the worst offenders—red dye 3—has since been banned from use in food (but not in cosmetics and other consumer products), several others may be just as toxic. Numerous studies find many of these dyes damage DNA in cells, suppress the immune system, can have neurotoxic effects (i.e., affect learning and memory), and lead to behavioral changes in children.

The CSPI's list also included what you might think of as an ingredient found only in Chinese food—monosodium glutamate. Check food labels; it's added to most processed foods to give them the taste of umami, considered the "fifth" taste after salty, sweet, sour, and bitter. Umami imparts a savory taste. Monosodium glutamate can cause flushing, headache, dizziness, heart palpitations, and nausea in some people.

And don't forget sodium nitrite, a salt used to preserve food and found in most smoked meats, hot dogs, and many deli meats. Nitrites appear to damage the genetic code in cells, leading to cancer-causing mutations. In fact, one study suggested they might be behind a recent increase in childhood brain tumors.

Another additive included on the original CSPI list and still found in many processed foods is butylated hydroxyanisole (BHA). Used to prevent fats, oils, and the foods that contain them from turning rancid, studies in rats show BHA can cause cancer. While the US Department of Health and Human Services classifies BHA as "reasonably anticipated to be a human carcinogen," the FDA still allows it in food.

Try Cutting Everything Out

One study of dietary chemical sensitivities in twenty-six people who had recurrent headaches found that the frequency and severity of headaches dropped in nearly all participants when they followed a diet with no monosodium glutamate, amines, tartrazine (yellow dye 5), preservatives, yeasts, nitrites/nitrates, or salicylate.

Even seemingly healthy food can be pumped up with toxins. Consider salmon, for instance. We're told to get more fish into our diets, that it's healthy for us. But 90 percent of the salmon in our grocery stores is farmed. Studies find that farm-raised salmon (and other fish) have much higher levels of PCBs (organic compounds used in manufacturing until they were banned in the 1970s) and dioxins (toxic by-products of manufacturing) than wild. Like pesticides, these poisons are considered POPs and accumulate in the fatty tissue of animals and humans.

Farmed salmon are also given synthetic chemicals to turn their skin pink so they look more like wild salmon (which get their pink color from naturally occurring carotenoids in the plants they eat). Since farm-raised salmon are brought up in such close quarters, disease is rampant and some farmers use massive amounts of antibiotics. The FDA has even blocked the sale of some farm-raised Chinese seafood because the fish were treated with antibiotics that are not allowed to be used on food animals in the United States. Meanwhile, some Canadian fish farmers use a pesticide banned in the United States to prevent sea lice infestation, which also occurs when fish are overcrowded.

When it comes to that hamburger you're eyeing, consider that it may contain one of six FDA-approved hormones, usually implanted into the animal from which the meat came. While the data on whether these hormones are dangerous to human health is mixed, it was enough for the European Agricultural Commission (EAC). In 1999, the EAC concluded that elevated levels of hormones in meat from implanted cattle might present a hazard, particularly to children. They had already been banned from use in food animals in Europe since 1989. The reality is that the additional hormones in our food supply represent one more thing your purification system has to deal with.

How about the water you drink? A 2005 study by the nonprofit Environmental Working Group found that the tap water in 42 states was contaminated with more than 140 unregulated chemicals, including MTBE, a gasoline additive; perchlorate, an ingredient used in rocket fuel that was spilled into groundwater during the Cold War; and industrial solvents. Drinking only bottled water doesn't protect you since much bottled water is really only tap water!

Drinking water in many communities also contains high amounts of arsenic, as does a lot of the red meat, chicken, and other poultry in our food supply. Arsenic is both a naturally occurring poison and a by-product of industrial processes. It's particularly prevalent in drinking water from wells.

One study published in the prestigious *Journal of the American Medical Association* found a strong link between urinary arsenic levels and diabetes. People with Type 2 diabetes—the most common type and the form that is now epidemic in our country—had arsenic levels 26 percent higher than those without diabetes. Overall, people with the highest blood levels of arsenic were nearly four times more likely to have diabetes than those with the smallest levels. Even people with levels low enough to

meet acceptable Environmental Protection Agency (EPA) stan-
dards were more likely to have diabetes.

Why the link? Researchers don't know for sure, but it may have
to do with the insulin-glucose partnership. Insulin is a hormone
produced in the pancreas that unlocks cells so they can receive
glucose, which they use for energy. When cells stop responding
to insulin in the bloodstream, they are said to be insulin resis-
tant. When this occurs, excess glucose and insulin build up in the
bloodstream. Too much can be toxic to certain cells and blood
vessels, leading to various diseases and medical conditions. Plus,
the high blood glucose levels signal the pancreas to keep churning out more insulin. Eventually, the insulin-producing cells in
the pancreas wear out and you have diabetes.

It seems that cells exposed to arsenic may be less reactive to
insulin. It also appears that arsenic may increase oxidative stress
and inflammation, which also contribute to diabetes.

Whenever you consume foods containing these toxins, your
body has to work all that much harder to get rid of them. And
even if you're a vegetarian or vegan, even if you're eating entirely
organic, you're still getting toxins from your food, the air, and
the environment.

Now, this is a lot of scary information being thrown at you,
but please believe us when we say we are *not* trying to convert
the masses into die-hard organic raw foodists. That doesn't even
describe us! Instead, we want to help you become better informed
about what you put into your body. But you have to live your life
and enjoy yourself: This is about finding the right balance.

Spending a few days drinking nothing but juices made from
organic fruits and vegetables dramatically cuts back on the
amount of toxins in your food supply. Plus, there's the added
bonus of giving your own detox system a much-needed rest.

Beware the Bottles of Bottled Water

If you've been buying bottled water to ensure a cleaner water supply, beware. The plastic often used to manufacture the bottles, as well as other food-related plastics such as storage containers for leftovers, contain a chemical called bisphenol A, which can leach out into food. Over time, studies suggest, this can lead to cancer, early puberty, and according to a recent study, may increase the risk of diabetes. Canada recently restricted the use of bisphenol A in food-related products, but in the summer of 2008 the FDA declared the chemical "safe" for its current uses.

Forget about bottled water when it comes to taking care of your body and reducing toxins. Purchase your own metal water bottle, keep it filled with filtered water, and carry it with you wherever you go. If you want your water cold, fill a couple halfway, freeze, and then fill with filtered water when you head out. The melting ice will keep the water cool for hours.

OUR FOOD ITSELF

Okay, so now you know about all the toxins in today's food supply. But what about the food itself? Why are we facing such an epidemic of obesity and diabetes in this country? Sure, we eat too much. But we also eat too much of the wrong things. We eat too many processed foods, too many foods filled with sugar and fat, too many foods that are so lacking in vitamins and minerals they have to be added, such as many breakfast cereals. (Total cereal is only "total" because of the added nutrients, not the nutrients inherent in the cereal itself.) Couple that with the high-stress lives we lead and watch the pounds pack on.

Yes, you heard us right: stress + high-fat/high-sugar diets = obesity. Stress has numerous effects on you physically. One such effect is the release of more glucose (energy) to fuel the "fight or flight" scenario that is the basis of all stress (even the stress related to your job). This increases your appetite, often sending you in search of high-fat/high-sugar foods that taste good and make you feel good. Stress also stimulates the release of chemicals that stimulate the growth of fat tissue.

This is particularly dangerous when it comes to the toxic world we live in, since many toxins accumulate in fat tissue. The more fatty tissue you have, the higher your toxic load.

This type of fat also tends to develop around abdominal organs such as your liver and pancreas, and around your waist. Then, in a kind of chicken-or-egg conundrum, the abdominal fat releases its own stress hormones, keeping the stress-eating-obesity cycle going and fueling inflammation, high cholesterol and blood insulin levels, glucose intolerance, high blood pressure, and "fatty" liver. Basically, stress makes people who are already overweight fatter.

Here then is yet another reason for the Cleanse. Our clients lose an average of two to three pounds on the 3-Day Cleanse, four to five on the 5-Day Cleanse, and six to seven on the 7-Day Cleanse. Some of that, hopefully, will come from abdominal fat. Plus, once you integrate cleansing into your life, you will find that you really can't handle the taste of fatty, sugary, and salty foods, and crave more natural foods both for your health and your taste buds. More of that abdominal fat will melt away, taking with it the toxins that can make you feel sluggish or even sick.

BETWEEN CLEANSES

Of course, you can't live on juices all the time. One of the best ways to detox is with a high-quality diet, which promotes healthy digestion. You know the drill: lots of fruits and vegetables, fresh foods not processed, etc. Here's how to get there in ten easy steps.

THE 3-DAY CLEANSE DETOX DIET

1. **Go organic when you can.** Yes, even organic fruits and vegetables may contain some pesticide residue resulting from the long-term poisoning of the soil in which they were grown, but the amounts are far less than what you would get with commercially grown produce. Yes, organic fruits and vegetables cost more than nonorganic produce. If you can't overhaul your entire grocery list at once, start with those items that are least protected from toxins: greens and fruits without skin or peels (strawberries and peaches should be at the top of your list of things to change).

2. **Go natural.** We're talking free-range chicken, beef, pork, lamb, and other meats raised on a natural diet without added hormones or antibiotics. And limit meat and poultry consumption to three ounces or less each time.

3. **Choose the right fish.** That would be wild fish. Yes, wild fish might cost more today (wild-caught salmon was $4-a-pound higher at our market than farmed salmon recently), but you'll save in the long run on health care costs! It's also important that you seek out fish that are low in mercury. Mercury is released as a by-product of coal burning and other industrial processes. Over the years it has penetrated nearly every waterway in the country and built up in the fatty tissue of certain fish.

   Fish highest in mercury include king mackerel, marlin, orange roughy, shark, swordfish, tilefish, tuna, and big eye ahi. So choose fish low in mercury, such as anchovies, catfish, shellfish, Atlantic croaker and haddock, herring, ocean perch, pollock, wild salmon, sardines, Pacific sole, tilapia, and freshwater trout. The Environmental Protection Agency and the Food and Drug Administration say that it is safe to eat most fish twice a week.

4. **Read labels.** Hate to have to throw in this one, but reading the *entire* label is a must. Because you cannot—repeat, *cannot*—take what a food package says at face value these days. Just because the box says "all-natural" doesn't mean what's inside it is. See page 17 for a list of some particularly loathsome additives.

5. **Shop the perimeter of the store.** If you stay on the perimeter, you're more likely to encounter single-ingredient foods: apples, milk, chicken, salmon—than if you head into the center aisles. These are foods untainted by preservatives, dyes, and flavorings. You can duck down an aisle for spices, pasta, dried beans, rice, etc. But stay away from items that are premade, frozen meals, "helpers" (e.g., Hamburger Helper), and foods loaded with sodium and sugar.

6. **Shop the health food section.** If you're lucky enough to have a good health food store near you (think Whole Foods or Trader Joe's), make it your first stop on grocery day. Even regular grocery stores now feature organic and health food sections. It might cost a little more in the short run to shop there, but trust us, it will be worth it in the long run!

7. **Stick to filtered, purified water.** Most filters that mount on your faucet or the top of your pitcher contain carbon as their primary filtering tool. Make sure that at the very least, your filter system is certified by NSF International—a nonprofit group that tests food and water products. The certification means that the filter can cleanse the water of all unwanted chemicals to the level set by the EPA. However, the resulting liquid may still contain some trace amounts of chemicals and these filters can't remove arsenic. Plus, replace the filter every couple of months or the filtering system is worthless.

If you're willing to spend the big bucks (sometimes

thousands of big bucks), consider a reverse-osmosis system, which uses a semipermeable membrane to remove contaminants. This type of system *can* remove arsenic and other metals.

8. **Eat as many raw foods as possible.** No matter how quickly it's done, by their very nature cooking and processing break down and reduce the amount of nutrients in fruits and vegetables. They also lead to significant loss of food-based enzymes that aid in digestion, putting more pressure on your internal digestive system.

9. **Skip the real *and* artificial sweeteners.** As we described earlier, chemical sweeteners may have a multitude of health-related effects, including high blood pressure, dizziness, and headaches. There's even some thought that saccharine—the main ingredient in the "pink" stuff—could be a culprit in inflammatory bowel disease, an autoimmune condition.

    Also skip foods with high-fructose corn syrup, a manufactured form of sweetener made from corn (most of it genetically engineered), which, studies find, prevent your brain from getting the proper signals that your stomach is full and you should stop eating. Some experts think high-fructose corn syrup may be a culprit in the obesity epidemic. Even "natural" sweeteners such as table sugar or molasses and honey can be toxic because the more sweet food you eat, the more sweet food you crave. Not only that, but studies find that fructose, whether natural (from fruit) or manufactured, can have the same effect on your liver as alcohol. Bottom line, if you *must* sweeten, you're better off doing so with real sugar than with any of the fake stuff. Our preference, however, is agave nectar, which you'll read more about later in the book.

10. **Aim for the whole thing.** We're talking whole grains, not refined. When manufacturers refine grains, they strip away the outer hull, in the process stripping away fiber, vitamins,

and minerals. In fact, most refined grains are then "fortified" by adding *back* minerals such as iron and vitamins such as niacin that have been stripped away. Whole grains are critical not only for good overall health, but for good digestion. In fact, they are critical for binding toxins in the small intestine so they can be escorted out of the body via feces. Not sure whether your "whole grain" bread is really whole grain? Here's a helpful hint: The words "whole wheat" should come first in the ingredients list.

In addition to changing your diet, you might want to check into other cleansing techniques that work well in conjunction with the 3-Day Cleanse. These approaches are particularly helpful for removing toxins that hide out in adipose tissue (i.e., fat).

- **A hard workout.** Exercise helps with detoxification in two ways. Physical activity itself increases blood flow through fat tissue, removing toxins for processing through the liver and kidneys, while sweating flushes out additional toxins from throughout your body. Just make sure you shower immediately after your workout to clean off those toxins before they can be reabsorbed.
- **Sauna.** Want to flush out your fat? Try a sauna. Although the sweating that occurs in a sauna is, in and of itself, detoxifying, studies also find that the heat from the sauna and its physiologic effects move toxins from fat tissue into the bloodstream, where they can be eliminated through the liver. Saunas also help detoxify by reducing oxidative stress, the cellular damage we talked about earlier. Sitting in a sauna even seems to increase your body's own ability to protect against oxidation. In fact, some doctors use it as part of a medical detoxification treatment, required when someone has been overexposed to some contaminants.

Just be careful not to stay in a sauna too long (15 to 20 minutes are usually the maximum recommended before taking a break) and finish up with a bottle of some water or, even better, green juice to replace the trace elements you lose through massive sweating. Also, skip the sauna if you have any heart-related issues, and save the alcoholic drinks for afterward (or better yet, skip the alcohol altogether to maximize the benefits of the detox).

- **Massage.** Massage, particularly deep-tissue or lymphatic massage, is another excellent way to break up toxins for removal. In deep-tissue massage, the therapist uses hands, knuckles, elbows—whatever it takes—against the grain on specific muscles to break up adhesions that cause pain and restrict movement. This focus on the stressed muscles also releases stored toxins. One study found that massage of the back, shoulder, head, and neck while in a seated position reduced symptoms of alcohol withdrawal in people going through detox. That's why it's so important that you drink lots of water after a massage to flush those toxins from your bloodstream.

   Lymphatic massage involves light, rhythmic strokes designed to improve the flow of lymph, a colorless fluid that runs throughout your body within its own network of glands and lymph vessels (more on the lymphatic system on page 28). Studies find that weekly lymphatic massages can really help move toxins through the lymphatic system for disposal.

- **Dry brush massage.** This is something you can do on your own; no massage therapist required! Simply take an all-natural shower brush (with soft bristles...not a loofah) and, starting at your feet and working your way up, firmly brush all areas of your skin. This removes dead skin cells, making room for new cells to form. It also revs up circulation, which is, after all, blood flow, helping to move toxins released during a Cleanse for removal.

- **Colonic hydrotherapy.** Yes, we're going to talk about it. While the 3-Day Cleanse will have a very...*cleansing* effect on your intestines, another approach to clear out that area is colon hydrotherapy. This technique pumps sterile, filtered water into the colon, prompting a bowel movement. People who are paralyzed and unable to move their own bowels use this approach, but these days even healthy people try an occasional colonic hydrotherapy for a kind of internal spring cleaning.

  There's also some thought that toxins leaking from the gut and bacteria moving from the gut to your bloodstream could lead to illness, particularly immune system malfunctions, so periodically detoxifying the colon might be a good idea. You can do your own colonic irrigation with any drugstore enema kit or with a colonic irrigation system, which requires a physician's prescription. If you choose to try the latter approach, find a therapist certified by and affiliated with the International Association of Colon Hydrotherapy (www.i-act.org; 210-366-2888). Also check with your state medical board—some states require licensure or certification for colonic irrigators. We can promise you that colonic cleansing is not gross or scary, even if it sounds that way. You won't believe how good you'll feel.

The Lymphatic System

If ever there were a body system that really got no respect, the lymphatic system would be it. A series of vessels, tissues, and organs, the lymphatic systems runs in the background, so to speak, of the circulatory system. It is responsible for returning fluid lost in tissues to the blood to maintain homeostasis, the balance that is so important to good health. The lymph nodes (found in the neck, under the arms, and in other parts of the body) help protect the body by removing foreign material such as bacteria and tumor cells and by providing a birthplace and resting ground for certain immune system cells. The dead material is sent back into the bloodstream for removal. Sometimes, however, large amounts of this toxic material can become clogged in the lymph nodes, leading to swelling and inflammation. Hence, the need for lymphatic massage.

A PEEK INSIDE

Now that you know why the food you eat and the life you live expose you to so many toxins and make the 3-Day Cleanse necessary, let's talk about how the internal workings of your body can benefit from the Cleanse.

Just how much do you know about what goes on inside you when you eat? How the food you eat becomes energy and feeds the cells and tissues of your body? Don't be embarrassed if your answer is "not much." Unless you're a die-hard nutritionist or a medical professional specializing in the gut and all its accoutrements, it's not something most of us think about.

So consider this your introduction to Digestion 101.

First, let's look at the main parts and their functions. We've even provided a picture on the next page (yeah, yeah, more than you wanted to know but there it is).

Digestion begins in your mouth. As you chew that steak dinner (grass-fed beef, of course), saliva released by tiny glands in your mouth both moistens your food and breaks it down via special enzymes. Before you know it, you've formed a glob of food called a *bolus*. Next thing you know, you've swallowed this

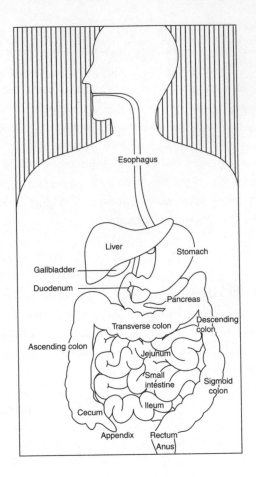

masticated mess and from then on what happens to it is out of your direct control.

What Is an Enzyme?

Throughout this book, you'll hear quite a bit about enzymes. So here's a good spot to explain them. An enzyme is an organic substance that acts as a catalyst to speed the rate of a chemical reaction without altering the reaction. Today we know of at least 700 different enzymes. Some work by accelerating the rate of breakdown through a substance's interaction with water; others accelerate oxidation reactions; and the third major type, called "reducing enzymes," remove oxygen from substances.

Enzymes perform a variety of jobs in your body, from speeding digestion to releasing energy so your heart can beat and your lungs expand and contract. They also digest cells after they die. For instance, the enzyme trypsin is used in medical treatments to clear out debris and dead tissue from wounds and burns.

Without enzymes, carbohydrates couldn't be turned into glucose or proteins into amino acids. Enzymes are also incredibly powerful; for instance, about one ounce of pepsin, the main enzyme found in stomach acid, can digest about a ton of egg whites (the purest protein known) in just a few hours.

The raw juices you drink during a Cleanse are chock full of highly potent enzymes that have not been killed through pasteurization. They are critical to the success of your Cleanse, and the reason why you must drink your juice as soon as you make it.

The journey from the mouth to, uh, the bathroom begins with the esophagus, a 10- to 13-inch tube that moves food not through gravity but through a series of muscular contractions weirdly similar to what happens when you squeeze sausage from its casing. Nice imagery, huh?

At the bottom of the esophagus a ring of muscle called a sphincter opens to let the bolus drop into the stomach. *Voilà!*

Your steak dinner has just arrived in digestion land. Here's where the real work begins. The stomach secretes gastric juice, a combination of a digestive enzyme called pepsin and an acid so strong that if some were to spill on you, it could eat through your clothing in no time.

All that acid serves two purposes: further breaking down your food and killing any bacteria or other nasty bugs that came in with the food (obviously, as recent food scares have shown, this is a less-than-perfect system). Anyway, after about two to six hours, that bolus is transformed into the lovely-sounding *chyme* and squirted through another muscular ring into the intestine like the proverbial you-know-what through a goose.

Two words about the intestine: 11 feet. That's how long this coiled tube that runs from the stomach to the anus would be if you took it out, hung it from a ceiling hook, and let it dangle down.

Okay, now that you've got *that* picture firmly embedded in your brain, let's move on. Once in the intestine, the chyme mixes with some more potent chemicals such as bile, which breaks down fat, pancreatic juice, and more enzymes. Lactase, for instance, breaks down lactose, a sugar found in milk and other unfermented dairy products (hence the phrase "lactose intolerant," which refers to your body's inability to produce enough lactase to break down lactose).

The chemicals the chyme encounters in the small intestine continue to break down the substance-formerly-known-as-food into molecular components such as glucose (sugar), amino acids (from the protein), and fatty acids (from the fat). These molecules glide through the intestinal wall into tiny blood vessels like ghosts moving through a haunted house. Then they travel through the bloodstream, where needy cells snatch them up.

Okay, back to the intestine. Unfortunately, not all of that

chyme can be broken down into nutritional molecules. The remainder moves into the large intestine, called the colon. It absorbs any water then holds the leftover chyme in its lower part (also called the bowel) for the following morning and your daily BM.

That smell in the bathroom? It's the result of bacteria called *E. coli* that the chyme picked up in the large intestine. These bacteria snack on some of the indigestible material left from the T-bone, in the process producing that stink. Interestingly, the less meat you eat, the less it smells because there's less indigestible material left over.

So there you are. Every morning (or afternoon or evening) when you go to the bathroom, you discharge a large amount of toxins from your body—all without your even being aware of the work that occurred to make it possible.

In the next chapter, we look at some of the science behind the 3-Day Cleanse and how it can help reduce illness and improve health.

Improve Your Digestion
(Beyond the 3-Day Cleanse)

The 3-Day Cleanse will improve your digestion. That's the top-line information you need to take away from this chapter. But as we said earlier, even *we* don't live on juice 24/7! So how can you improve your digestion when you're *not* cleansing? Read on.

1. Follow the right kind of diet. We believe very strongly in a mostly raw, mostly vegetarian diet eaten along the principles of "food combining." Food combining is a way of eating that recognizes that different enzymes are responsible for breaking down different foods. Therefore, you try not to mix certain foods that require different enzymes and that are broken down at different rates. We will explain all this in *much* more detail in Chapter 7, but for now, we ask that you keep an open mind about it. Eating this way enables your digestive system to work in a more structured, organized manner, reducing that overstuffed, bloated feeling common with the typical American diet. With food combining, eating becomes less about what you're eating and more about how and when you're eating, so you can still indulge in certain things you might otherwise feel you'd need to eliminate.

2. Stay active. If you're constipated, chances are the first thing your doctor will ask is, "Are you exercising?" You simply cannot expect things to work as they should if the only movement you get is from your desk or your couch to the kitchen or bathroom! You have to get out there and *move* if you want to keep everything inside, ah…moving! We're not talking 26-mile marathons here. A 30-minute walk every day should help immensely. And don't discount "nonexercise" exercise like dancing, yard work, cleaning your house, washing your car, and even sex. They all involve twisting and moving your body, increase oxygen intake, and induce you to drink more liquids—all of which will help with digestion.

3. Say *ohhmmm*. Yoga, Pilates, or other movement-based programs that use a combination of stretching and deep breathing to strengthen muscles and improve blood flow are ideal for digestion. They are also known stress relievers, which is critically important to good digestion. Believe it or not, your gut contains some of the same mood-related hormones as your brain, particularly serotonin. In fact, some consider the gut a second brain. That's why you get butterflies in your stomach when you're nervous, can't eat or go to the bathroom when you're stressed, or get diarrhea when you're upset. Also, when you're stressed, your body releases stress hormones that, basically, shunt blood away from the stomach to other parts of the body such as the heart and lungs. Without a good blood supply, digestion slows.

4. Get the kinks worked out. We talked about the benefits of massage for detoxing. But how about for improving digestion? Studies find massage can improve appetite and digestion in premature infants and relieve constipation in adults with irritable bowel syndrome. Imagine the benefits for someone who simply needs improved digestion! Treat yourself to at least a monthly massage and make sure to share with your therapist your goal of improved digestion.

5. Learn to chill. As noted, one reason yoga and Pilates are so effective at improving digestion is that they have strong stress-relieving properties. They are not, however, the only way to go about managing your stress. Yes, we said "managing" your stress, not eliminating it. You can't eliminate stress in your life, nor should you. Think how boring (and stressful) your life would be if everything were as bland as a rice cake. Plus, even good events can be stressful (think about a wedding, a new baby, or buying a new home).

What you *can* do, however, is learn to better cope with that stress. And that's important, because when you're under stress, whether acute—getting a flat tire—or chronic—coping with a serious illness in your family—your body releases various hormones that affect nearly every physiologic system. Your heart speeds up, you take in more oxygen, your liver releases more glucose for energy, and your pancreas floods your body with insulin to move that glucose into cells. All of which creates a significant amount of inflammation and results in the formation of those nasty free radicals. So the idea is to remain calm when you're stressed, thus dampening that hormonal response. Some of our favorite ways (beyond a dirty martini) include:

- **Deep breathing.** Few of us know how to breathe properly. We are too likely to take quick shallow breaths that do nothing in terms of providing the full amount of oxygen our body needs not only for detoxing but also for digestion. No matter where you are or what you're doing, find a moment to take a few deep breaths. That means breathing in through your nose and not stopping until you see your stomach and diaphragm rise; and out through your nose, not stopping until you can feel no more air in your lungs. Do this ten times.
- **Give yourself a time-out.** We do it to our children; we all had it done to us when we were kids. Take five minutes and go for a walk, close your eyes, remove yourself from the situation. This is possibly the most effective way to chill out.

CHAPTER 2

Beyond the Hype:
What the Science Shows

Hello! Just had to write and share something with you guys: I did a three-day juice fast with you last week. At the same time, my sixty-five-year-old mother was being discharged from the hospital after emergency intestinal surgery, during which she had not eaten solid food for ten days. The surgeon mandated a low-fiber diet to start but the only thing on his list of thirty foods that Mom was able to get down was chicken broth, and then only with tremendous difficulty. I shared some of my green juice from the Cleanse with her and she loved it. So, because of you she was able to get nourishment not otherwise available. I'm sure it's helping her heal.
— MARYLIN, A BLUEPRINTCLEANSE CLIENT

I'm stunned at the amount of energy I have, the clarity with which I'm able to think, and, mostly, the realization of how much garbage I was putting into my system. There are several people in my office who have commented that I actually look healthier. Thanks so much. I truly feel like this is one of those moments in my life that I will never forget because of the impact it has and will continue to have on my health.
— PAUL, A BLUEPRINTCLEANSE CLIENT

Yes, we told you in Chapter 1 that the Cleanse is not a fast. But it *is* based on the underlying philosophy of a fast, which is, in and of itself, a cleansing. Thus, we devote this chapter to explaining the history, symbolism, and physiology (i.e., how it works in your body) of fasting. We also throw in some benefits that might surprise you, benefits based not just on our experience, but on actual medical studies.

Although fasting can trace its roots back thousands of years—likely to the first cave dwellers who suggested that a day without food might help appease the gods that just burned down their forest and decimated their bison herd—it still maintains a remarkably modern role.

Then, as now, fasting was viewed as a spiritual step, a way to bring yourself closer to said "gods," to strip yourself of all distractions, to cleanse (!) and purify as a way of becoming one with the universe. As Saint Augustine said of fasting: "It cleanses the mind, raises the soul." Of course, the fact that a brain without glucose is a brain likely to hallucinate (aka see visions) probably didn't hurt either.

The Judeo-Christian religions embraced the pagan ritual of fasting. The Bible, for instance, mentions fasting throughout. Even today, Jews fast on Yom Kippur, the Day of Atonement, to beg forgiveness for their sins. Christian religions embrace fasting during Lent, fasting on Ash Wednesday and Good Friday, but "giving up" something as penance for the remainder of the forty days. Even the Catholic tradition of meatless Fridays evokes a wisp of the fast. And why do you think Ash Wednesday is preceded by "Fat Tuesday" and Mardi Gras, when consumption of alcohol and rich foods peaks? Think of it as religion's own form of "cleansing."

FASTING FOR HEALTH

I started juicing because I knew my body was not at optimal health. I have nothing serious, but at times I've experienced too much fatigue, bloating, constipation, joint pain, a general malaise. Juicing definitely clears up all these symptoms and in a very short time.

—RACHEL

The first reports of fasting for medical reasons date back to the early 1800s. "Every disease that afflicts mankind [comes from] more or less habitual eating in excess of the supply of gastric juices," wrote a leading physician of the time, Edward Hooker Dewey, M.D., in his book *The True Science of Living*. Dewey, who also opposed breakfast, wrote: "Take away food from a sick man's stomach and you have begun, not to starve the sick man, but the disease."

As you might imagine, fasting has long been a preferred option for losing weight. As early as 1915 doctors recommended repeated yet short incidences of fasting for weight loss, particularly in very overweight people. One paper published in the early 1960s detailed the weight loss of 107 people who fasted under medical supervision for 14 days. Overall, participants lost an average of two to three pounds a day. Generally, by the second day people they stopped feeling hungry (something you'll also notice on the Cleanse). Three people with terrible psoriasis, an autoimmune skin disease that causes awful itching and rashes, found their skin completely cleared during the fast. In addition, several people with hypertension had normal blood pressure by the fast's end. Perhaps the most amazing results came from the fact that even 32 months after the fast ended, 43 of the participants maintained their weight loss and 17 percent continued to lose. You don't see those statistics even with traditional diets!

More recently, the prestigious *New England Journal of Medicine* wrote: "Fasting is a valid experience. It can benefit any otherwise healthy person whose calories now have the upper hand in his/her life."

We are certainly not recommending a fast—or even a Cleanse—for weeks at a time. But the benefits of the occasional day or week without food can really be amazing. And while you may be doing the Cleanse just to feel better after a bit too much eggnog and stuffing during the holidays, or to drop a few pounds before your high school reunion, it's worth paying attention to the long-term benefits of fasting and cleansing, as well. Here's what the medical evidence shows:

- **Heart disease.** Question: Why do people who live in Utah have one of the lowest rates of death from heart disease in the United States? Answer: Most are Mormon and so don't smoke, ingest caffeine, drink, or engage in other unhealthy behaviors. But, asked researchers from the University of Utah in Salt Lake City, could there be something else at work? Something like the fasting the Mormons do once a month? To find out, they compared the heart health of about 4,600 Utah residents with various lifestyle factors, including fasting. They found that people who fasted on average once a month (whether Mormon or not) were 77 percent less likely to have coronary artery disease (a buildup of plaque and gunk along artery walls that leads to heart attack and stroke) than people who never fasted. That improvement held even after the researchers controlled for weight, blood pressure, cholesterol levels, age, diabetes, smoking, and family history—all major risk factors for heart disease.

So what's going on? One theory is that anyone who is self-disciplined enough to fast once a month is probably also self-disciplined enough to follow a healthy diet and exercise regularly, which also reduces the risk of heart disease. That sounds nice, but the docs think the real reason lies in the effects of periodic fasting in insulin and glucose sensitivity.

Remember in the previous chapter when we talked about insulin sensitivity and how insulin resistance—when your cells turn their proverbial backs on insulin and refuse to allow the hormone to unlock their doors to glucose—is behind numerous chronic health conditions as well as weight gain? Well, it turns out that periodic fasting seems to "reboot" the whole insulin-glucose system.

Skip eating for a few days and your pancreas (the insulin-producing factory) becomes more responsive to signals from other parts of your body that glucose is needed, while cells that use glucose, such as muscle cells, become more sensitive to insulin. *Voilà!* No insulin resistance—which we now know is a major contributor to heart disease.

- **Diabetes.** As you might expect, if you're doing better at getting insulin and glucose onto and into cells, you're less likely to get diabetes. That's just what those University of Utah researchers found in the study described earlier. Just 11 percent of the Utah natives they studied who already *had* moderate heart disease, but who periodically fasted, also had diabetes. Compare that to the people with heart disease who *didn't* fast, 20 percent of whom had diabetes. The benefits worked both ways. Participants *with* diabetes who fasted were also far less likely to have heart disease than those with diabetes who didn't fast. This is really important since people with diabetes are twice as likely to have a heart attack or stroke as someone without diabetes.

- **Learning and memory.** At least two studies find that restricting calories about 30 percent (but no lower than 1,200 calories a day) improves memory, verbal ability, and other cognitive functions. The reason? Possibly reduced inflammation, which leaves brain cells healthier and better able to do their job of processing information.
- **Asthma.** Speaking of reduced inflammation, a study involving ten people with asthma found those who reduced their calories to near fasting levels (about 350 calories) every *other* day for two months had fewer asthma symptoms and better lung function than those who didn't. They also showed fewer signs of inflammation and oxidative stress, both key contributors to asthma. They also dropped about 8 percent of their body weight!
- **Weight loss.** Here's the news you've been waiting for. Those Utah study participants who fasted once a month or so were far less likely to be overweight than those who didn't fast. More about weight loss later in this chapter.

What's important about all this, and what we want you to keep in mind as you move through the rest of the book and begin your own Cleanse, is that none of these studies involved people who were fasting for a week at a time. Some weren't even fasting, just reducing their calories. Even the Mormons define "fasting" as "not eating or drinking for two consecutive meals."

So just imagine what the short- *and* long-term benefits of cleansing for three days every month could be. Yeah, pretty amazing, huh?

Just listen to what physicians say about the benefits of fasting.

One of the earliest to embrace fasting for health was Otto Buchinger, Sr., M.D., a German physician who founded several clinics in which he conducted more than 100,000 "juice fasting cures." "Juice fasting is, without any doubt, the most effective biological method of treatment," he wrote. "It is the 'operation without surgery'...it is a cure involving exudation, reattunement, redirection, loosening up and purified relaxation."

As Dr. James Balch and his wife, Carol, both proponents of natural healing and the authors of several books on the topic, have noted: "Fasting is an effective and safe method of detoxifying the body...A technique that wise men have used for centuries to heal the sick. Fast regularly and help the body heal itself and stay well. Give all of your organs a rest. Fasting can help reverse the aging process, and if we use it correctly we will live longer, happier lives."

Meanwhile, Joel Fuhrman, M.D., author of *Eat for Health*, *Eat to Live*, *Cholesterol Protection*, and other nutritional books, says that in his practice, "I have seen fasting eliminate lupus and arthritis, remove chronic skin conditions such as psoriasis and eczema, heal the digestive tract in patients with ulcerative colitis and Crohn's disease, and quickly eliminate cardiovascular diseases such as high blood pressure and angina. In these cases the recoveries were permanent."

And as we said before, fasting doesn't have to mean a water-only diet. Rudolph Ballentine, M.D., who established holistic medical clinics in Chicago, New York, Buffalo, Pittsburgh, Minneapolis, and Honesdale, Pennsylvania, and authored *Radical Healing: Integrating the World's Great Therapeutic Traditions to Create a New Transformative Medicine*, says the "ideal technique" for successful fasting is using fresh, raw fruit and vegetable juices. "On such a diet, the full spectrum of nutrients is supplied in an easily assimilated form, so the digestive tract is able to remain essentially at rest."

And Gabriel Cousens, M.D., who founded and runs the Tree of Life Rejuvenation Center in Patagonia, Arizona, where hundreds of people a year come to fast, says he finds that after four days of fasting, his clients report improved concentration, expanded creative thinking, and a lifting of their depression. "Insomnia stops, anxieties fade, the mind becomes more tranquil, and a natural joy begins to appear. It is my hypothesis that when the physical toxins are cleared from the brain cells, mind-brain function automatically and significantly improves and spiritual capacities expand."

One doctor, Rai Casey, M.D., supervised hundreds of fasts as a physician with a New York City medical practice. "I found that the physical healing or weight loss was but a pleasant side effect. What really happened is that the person got in touch with their higher self, their true self, and came to the experience that healing can take place at every level, simply by letting go and allowing Mother Nature to do her work."

Finally, one of the fathers of modern fasting, Herbert M. Shelton, D.C., N.D., who wrote *The Science and Fine Art of Fasting,* says that "fasting must be recognized as a fundamental and radical process that is older than any other mode of caring for the sick organism, for it is employed on the plane of instinct and has been employed since life was first introduced upon the earth. Fasting is nature's own method of ridding the body of 'diseased tissues,' excess nutriment and accumulations of waste and toxins. Nothing else will increase elimination through every channel of excretion as will fasting."

Of course, we enjoy hearing from our clients about what they perceive as the benefits of cleansing. Here's what Sydney, sixty-six, had to say about juice cleansing and why she does it: "I do a juice fast every quarter, sometimes more often. I'm sixty-six and in great shape, especially compared to a lot of my contemporaries, who moan and whine about how awful they feel. At the same time, most of them won't listen to any advice about ways to change their situation. I don't mean to sound unkind. I'm just impatient with this notion of 'It's just old age and there's nothing I can do about it.' Nonsense!"

Rebooting Your Taste Buds

You are right. All I want are healthy things. No thoughts of a martini, returning to my huge mug of morning coffee, or even whole wheat pasta have crossed my mind.

—Nathalie, a BluePrintCleanse client

Maybe you've always considered yourself a sugaraholic. Or figured that a meal without a saltshaker nearby is not worth eating. Well, get ready to change your perception of yourself.

Here's the thing. Your taste buds are more malleable than a handful of Silly Putty. Go just twenty-four hours without sugar, fat, or salt (SFS), and you'll immediately notice a difference in how those ingredients taste. Extend that SFS fast for three, five, or seven days (as with a Cleanse) and it's like wiping clean the hard drive of your taste buds. Suddenly, that burger tastes like it was dipped in grease; the fries taste so salty you'd swear someone dumped the entire shaker on them; and the shake feels like the waitress added a cup of confectioners' sugar just for kicks. Yet pre-Cleanse you would have gobbled them up and asked for more.

Here's where two important benefits of the Cleanse come in. Not only will periodic Cleanses "reboot" your taste buds to enjoy healthier fare and shun SFS, but because you now prefer healthier fare and shun most SFS, those pounds you lost during the Cleanse can stay lost.

FASTING TO LIVE LONGER

Here's an unexpected benefit you might find once you begin cleansing and living the Cleansing Life: a longer life.

Yup, you heard us right. Cut back on the calories overall and you could add years to your life. And these would be good years, relatively free of disease and infirmity.

One of the most exciting areas of research right now is on the benefits of calorie restriction. We're not talking about slashing your calories in half, but cutting them 15 to 25 percent. So if you're used to eating about 2,000 calories a day, skip dessert, give up the frozen mocha latte, and switch from whole milk to skim. Six hundred or so calories just went missing.

Studies find reducing calories can increase longevity in numerous animal models, including worms and fruit flies. Studies are currently ongoing on the effects on mammals, including humans, but savvy researchers have already found several health benefits, including many covered earlier.

The experts don't know exactly *why* calorie restriction works such magic, but they do have some theories. One is that if you're not eating as much, your body doesn't have to expend as much energy breaking down food (refer back to Chapter 1 if you don't think it takes a lot of energy to break down food). Remember what happens when you digest food that cells then pull in to create energy? Remember what happens when cells make energy? They create lots of free radicals. Recall our formula: free radicals = inflammation = cell damage. Cell damage = aging, disease, weight gain, and just feeling plain awful.

Another theory suggests that intermittent fasting, which leads to overall calorie reduction similar to what occurs when you periodically cleanse, stresses cells just enough so they become stronger overall, sort of the way that lifting weights creates tiny tears in muscles that, once they heal, make for a stronger muscle.

Researchers have also found that fasting every couple of weeks or so slows cell turnover. Cells don't divide as often, reducing the risk of errors that can lead to diseases such as cancer.

We figure a monthly 3-Day Cleanse trims more than 3,000 calories a month from your diet. Although there's no way to really know if it will help you live longer, the science is on your side!

MORE ABOUT WEIGHT LOSS

Here's the thing about the Cleanse. People who do it want to appear as if they're doing it for only the purest of reasons. Their overall health; to give their detox organs a rest; to reduce their risk of disease, hasten recovery from disease, or simply feel better.

But we know the *real* reason you're cleansing: *to lose weight*.

Don't be embarrassed! We're on your side! In fact, we'd bet most of our clients are on the weight-loss side of the equation. Because the thing is, the Cleanse can be a healthy way to drop a few pounds *fast*.

The first day, your body burns stored glucose called glycogen for energy. By the second day, however, that glycogen is gone and your body starts breaking down fat for energy. This, of course, releases all those stored toxins we talked about in the previous chapter, sending them into the bloodstream, where they can be filtered by the liver and kidneys and excreted.

Studies of people who fast show that in the first few days, normal weight people can expect to lose about two pounds a day. If you're overweight, expect that figure to be higher. More isn't better, however. The longer you fast or cleanse, the less weight you'll lose. That's because after a while, your body figures out what's going on and clamps down on every molecule of fat. This is why diets fail so miserably, particularly cyclical dieting. The more you diet, the more your body learns to slow its metabolism at the first sign of a food scale.

No worries with the Cleanse; even a 7-Day Cleanse won't affect your long-term ability to drop the pounds or slow your metabolism because you cleanse for only a few days at a time, too short a time to change your overall metabolism. Also, because you're still getting about 1,200 calories a day, you are not "starving" your body, so there is no reason for it to slow the rate at which it burns those calories.

Wait…we can hear you now. "But isn't that weight loss just

water?" We've never really understood what this means. Yes, you will find that you're peeing a lot while on the Cleanse, possibly every hour if you're taking in enough filtered water and teas. This is really important to help flush out those toxins. But you're not losing water weight. When the weight is lost, it's from the fat that gets burned to maintain equilibrium between energy in and energy out.

The reality is that while you're getting about 1,200 calories or less per day during a Cleanse, your typical diet is probably twice that. Another difference between the Cleanse and a "diet" is that you won't be hungry. The ingredients in the juices are designed not just for weight loss but also for detoxing. Because they provide maximum nutrients and because your taste buds change during the Cleanse, you are less likely to return to your old eating habits and thus more likely to keep the weight off.

We don't, however, recommend doing a Cleanse for weight-loss reasons only. If you return to your regular eating habits, the weight *will* return. Our hope is that you find the benefits of the Cleanse so empowering that you decide to change the way you eat all the time, hopefully with our recommendations in Chapter 7 about food combining and building more of your diet around raw foods.

SOME CONCLUDING WORDS

The best thing about cleansing? Feeling clean, light, free, healthy...no more cravings; feeling very connected to myself and to life and to divine inspiration.

The worst thing about cleansing? Feeling hungry for the first couple of days, fantasizing about what I'll eat when I'm off the fast, occasional fatigue or weakness, having to break the Cleanse (at some point it gets easier to just keep cleansing!).

—KIRA

If we haven't convinced you that cleansing is a great way to drop a few pounds, clear out accumulated toxins, and reboot your taste buds, not to mention improve your overall health, then we've failed. But we're pretty sure that by now you're raring to put the book down and either call us for the BluePrintCleanse ready-made juices or head into the kitchen to make your own.

We're excited that you're excited! But slow down just a bit. First, you have to decide which Cleanse is best for you and identify your own goals for cleansing, all of which we cover in the next chapter.

CHAPTER 3

Choosing the Cleansing Option That's Right for You

Okay, now we get to the nitty gritty of your Cleanse. And we mean *your* Cleanse, not your mother's Cleanse, or your boyfriend's Cleanse, or your best friend's Cleanse. For the Cleanse that's right for them is not necessarily the Cleanse that's right for you. In fact, the Cleanse that's right for you *today* may not be the Cleanse that's right for you next month or next year.

Unlike other juice cleanses or fasts, our Cleanse is not a one-size-fits-all program. We designed it around three levels because we understand that everyone has different needs and tolerance levels, i.e., different needs for cleansing and different abilities to tolerate the process.

We realized that if cleansing was to be truly effective and something people *wanted* to do (and do often), it had to be more than just a single, unforgiving process for everyone regardless of their individual habits.

Enter the three levels. We've customized each of the three Cleanses so you can pick and choose based on your individual needs and personal schedule. For instance, maybe after the holidays or a major binge (ten days of all-you-can-eat buffets on a Caribbean cruise comes to mind), you opt for the Level 3 Excavation Cleanse for five days.

But maybe every month as ongoing maintenance you pencil in a Level 1 Cleanse for three days. The key here is flexibility.

The only thing we recommend is that you start with a Level 1 Cleanse if this is your first-ever Cleanse. Level 1 has more fruit juices than green juices, so for many people, it simply tastes better. It also has the highest calories (about 1,200), so you're less likely to feel any kind of weakness. We also recommend starting with a 3-Day Cleanse. Not only will it get the cleansing process off to a good start and do far more in terms of cleaning out the dark places than a 1- or 2-Day Cleanse, but it will help you understand the importance of the pre-Cleanse preparation (more on that in Chapter 4) and the post-Cleanse reentry (more on that in Chapter 6).

However, even a 1-Day Cleanse is beneficial. As one client wrote on her blog: "My advice for those considering the Cleanse who haven't juiced before: If you haven't juiced before, start with the one-day program. The first day was the most manageable for me. I already saw the benefits of a flatter stomach and increased energy after one day. If you opt for a three-day or longer program, don't beat yourself up. Even after I cheated, I still felt really good and healthy when I drank the next juice."

We recommend a 3-Day Cleanse to start, but if you're going to ease into it with just a 1-Day Cleanse, make sure you are *very* diligent when you prepare and on the first day after the Cleanse.

Once you've completed your first Cleanse and see how amazing you feel, then you can move on to the more intensive Cleanses or, conversely, stick with Level 1 for fewer or more days. We even had an Excavation Cleanser (the most intense level) transition at the end of his Cleanse not to solid food, but to the second level, followed by the first level, and then eventually reincorporate solid foods again until he resumed his normal diet. Here's an important message for you: More is *not* necessarily better. Here in America we tend to think that if a little is good, a lot is better.

Not always. Too much of anything can be dangerous. You can decide how long you want to go but we generally recommend three to fourteen days.

If you're considering an extended Cleanse it is even more critical to make sure you take the proper measures to clean out the huge amounts of toxins that will be released, such as colonics (more on these on page 28). Otherwise, your body will reabsorb those toxins and you won't get the full benefits of the extended Cleanse. Another thing that is important is to practice proper dental hygiene—not just by flossing and brushing, but by chewing a raw carrot or apple once a day to further clean your teeth.

Now, having said that, we don't want you to feel that if you can't handle a Level 2 or Level 3 Cleanse, or if you can't make it past Day 2 on any level Cleanse, that you have somehow failed or will lose out on the benefits.

No way! Any Cleanse is a good Cleanse. The key is listening to your body. The 3-Day Cleanse is a tool. Use as needed.

WHEN TO CLEANSE?

Well, that's a good question. We like to think of Cleanses in two ways: the regular, maintenance Cleanse that you should do once a month, and the "I've done too much tied one on can't get myself together" Cleanse you should do as needed. Here's how we view them.

Think of the maintenance Cleanse as a kind of oil change for your body. Just as you change the oil in your car every 3,000 miles or so, you need to change the "oil" in your body every four weeks or so. By oil we mean fuel, the fuel that feeds every cell and builds every tissue. For three days (more or less if you like, but most of our clients do 3-Day Cleanses), you switch out the hamburger-fries-wine-beer-martini-pizza-soda diet for one filled with some of the healthiest ingredients your poor cells have ever encountered.

We get it. It's hard to eat nine servings of fruits and vegetables every day. But for every day you're on the Cleanse, you'll be getting more than that every day. The benefits are tremendous, as you'll see later in this chapter when we describe the specific ingredients in your cleansing juices.

Then there's the second kind of Cleanse. The kind of Cleanse you do once your New Year's Eve hangover dissipates. When you return from that week in Aruba. After the excesses of Thanksgiving—or after a really rough month at work during which you lived on fast food, five hours of sleep, superstrong coffee, and Red Bull. When you need to hit the reset button.

When to Cleanse?

Here's what some of our clients tell us about when they choose to cleanse:

- I cleanse when I need to "clean up" my diet after some transgressions (vacations, holidays, overworking, etc.) and when I feel aches and pains or a cold coming on. One or two days of juice fasting and I never get sick!
- I like to cleanse every Monday—it's like a safety net for my health! It's also easy because I know I don't have to spend time cooking or eating. It's like a vacation for the body, mind, and spirit!
- I like to cleanse when the seasons change, especially from summer to fall and winter to spring. I usually do a 7-Day Cleanse to signal the internal changes that go along with the change of seasons. And I focus on foods that are grown in season (beets in the fall, asparagus in the spring).

Here's why Suzi cleanses: "I am a restaurant/dining writer and social columnist and my boyfriend owns several restaurants.

I go out to dinners and parties about six nights a week and I'm always eating heavy gourmet food and drinking wine. I need these Cleanses to press the reset button on my eating habits every once in a while!"

Her first Cleanse came about because she felt "toxic." "I was so hooked on nonfat this and that, and so many chemical-ridden food items, that one day it just clicked: I need an intervention!"

The intervention, of course, was the 3-Day Cleanse.

Cleanse Clients Ask . . .
How long should I cleanse?
Depends on you. Different Cleanses accomplish different things. A 3-Day Cleanse helps your body clear out the dregs, stuff that's been hanging out there for a while. A 5-Day Cleanse begins the rebuilding and healing process, while a 10-Day Cleanse may provide protection against long-term, chronic disease. While the focus of this book is the 3-Day Cleanse, we will provide guidelines for the 1-Day, 5-Day, and 10-Day as well.

Even a 1-Day Cleanse can be fabulous, and we have clients who do the 1-Day Cleanse once a week. A 1-Day Cleanse done regularly is a great way to give your body a quick rest, strengthen your immune system during cold/flu season, or sharpen mental clarity. It's a time-out, a break, a way of allowing your body to catch up.

While the cleansing length is a personal decision, you will feel different depending on how long you cleanse for. After all, just two extra days (when you go from a 3- to a 5-Day Cleanse) means 60 percent more cleansing time! That means 60 percent more detoxing!

CHOOSE YOUR LEVEL

Okay, now we get to the part where you choose your level. We've given personalities to our levels (makes them so much more personal and fun). As you work through the information in the levels and the quiz that begins on page 66, remember that the level you choose is less a matter of what you *need*, and more a matter of which level is right for you *at this time.* What are you most comfortable doing? What level do you think you can manage best?

Also keep in mind that the level you are today is not necessarily the level you'll be the next time you cleanse. Plus, you don't have to go through your levels in order; in other words, just because you did a Level 3 Cleanse last time doesn't mean that's the level you need to do on your next Cleanse. It's fine to revisit the Level 1 Renovation Cleanse at any time.

THE RENOVATION CLEANSE

We (and our clients) call this the "Gateway Cleanse." It encourages you to move on to the next two levels of the 3-Day Cleanse and, well, you will find how it makes you feel to be quite addictive.

You Know You're a Renovation Cleanser If...

- You figure the lettuce, tomato, and ketchup on your burger equates to three servings of vegetables.
- You consider "whole foods" to be those that don't need to be cut up, like chicken nuggets.
- Your favorite vegetable is French fries.
- Your favorite fruit is whatever is garnishing the cocktail in your hand.

- You consider a day without Pinot Noir to be a very bad day, indeed.
- Your idea of eating healthier is to buy the free-range hamburger instead of the regular stuff.

The Renovation Cleanse places you on the path to feeling and looking better. This Cleanse is designed for the absolute beginner—the "I'll have my martini with a side of steak, please" type. Our Renovators are the ones who could stand to lose a few pounds (or maybe even more than a few, but who's counting?).

You tend to indulge, sometimes in excess...a few extra drinks here...a side of onion rings there...maybe you even sneak in the occasional (or not so occasional) cigarette. Doesn't matter. You are about to experience one of the greatest changes in your life. This level has just enough calories to curb any unpleasant side effects such as headaches, dizziness, and nausea. So you can still go about your daily life while simultaneously giving your insides a breather.

On this Cleanse you'll feel more energetic, find your moods stabilizing, and be more productive. When you finish, expect compliments. "Did you lose weight?" "What kind of moisturizer are you using? Your skin looks amazing!"

This level also contains the highest amount of fruit in the juices, so the juices themselves taste sweeter, making them more palatable for people just beginning to cleanse. On the Renovation Cleanse, you drink six juices a day: two green juices, three fruit juices, and one nut milk. The recipes begin on page 135. Which ones you choose is entirely up to you!

THE FOUNDATION CLEANSE

Our Foundation types are active, busy people who exercise and try to eat healthy, but can't always get their hands on fresh, whole foods (not every town has a health food store on every corner like Manhattan!) or simply don't have the time to mess with it. So even though you try to eat right and live the healthy life, you often get that bloated, sluggish feeling as a result of slipping.

Too much processed food. Too much white flour. Too many Christmas cookies, a glass of wine that turned into a bottle, the fast-food salad that somehow morphed into the double cheese-burger. Trust us, we've been there!

Unlike Renovators, who are typically completely oblivious to what they put in their system (or are aware of how poor their habits are), a Founder makes the effort to be healthy, but probably not often enough. Maybe you're a vegetarian but eat more dairy than you should. Maybe you eat brown rice and whole grains, but in combination with heavy, dense protein such as steak or chicken. Or maybe you eat a *lot* of soy products, thinking it's healthy when, in fact, too much soy can expose your body to too much protein and too many plant-based hormones that resemble estrogen. A Founder might be someone who exercises four times in one week followed by once the next week, and who enjoys organic foods paired with a vodka martini.

The Foundation Cleanse will take care of those warning signs you've been feeling, the sense that something just isn't right. You know…afternoon headache, trouble falling asleep (and staying asleep), mysterious aches and pains that make you feel about thirty years older than you are.

You Know You're a Foundation Cleanser If...

- You *want* to be a vegetarian but just can't give up the lamb lollipop.
- You always order a large salad at lunch—with the chicken, bleu cheese, and crunchy noodles.
- You belong to a gym; you just don't go.
- You keep three pairs of jeans in your closet: skinny, normal, and "what the hell have I been eating?"
- You always order fruit for dessert...with the cheesecake underneath.
- Your pantry is filled with beans, whole wheat pasta, quinoa, and Israeli couscous, but your freezer is filled with vodka.

The Foundation Cleanse also contains six juices a day: three green juices, two fruit juices, and one nut milk.

THE EXCAVATION CLEANSE

The Excavation Cleanse is our most intense Cleanse. It is not something you go into lightly! This Cleanse gives your system a serious rest. We recommend it only for serious cleansers. While on Level 3, you might find a part of yourself you haven't seen in years or didn't even know existed. You will literally be turning yourself inside out to find the "you" that you've known was there all along. Don't start on this level unless you've worked your way up to it, or scored a 20 or more on the quiz on page 66. Otherwise, it might be too overwhelming and could turn you off to cleansing altogether, something that doesn't do anyone any good! Excavation differs from the other two levels in that it has about 400 fewer calories than Level 1, and 200 fewer calories than Level 2 (but who's counting?). Most important, however, is that it contains the highest number of green juices and, thus, the greatest amount of alkalizing vegetables designed to bring the pH of your blood into balance. On the Excavation Cleanse you drink four green juices, one fruit juice, and one nut milk.

The additional benefit you get from the increased chlorophyll from the plants is very important. Studies find that chlorophyll has amazing healing properties, even helping cancer patients escape many side effects from chemotherapy.

The Excavation Cleanse is our most intense. More often than not, our Excavators tend to go for a longer Cleanse, often six or ten days.

You Know You're an Excavation Cleanser If...

- Your daily, two-hour workout at the gym takes precedence over dinner with your best friend.
- The last time you ate cooked food was when you hiked the Appalachian Trail.
- You chase your organic cocktail with a shot of wheatgrass.
- Your favorite mode of transportation (other than your own two feet) is transcendental meditation.
- You're a breath away from breathitarian.
- You cleanse not because you normally follow a mediocre diet, but because you need to detox from twenty-first-century living.

SAMPLE CLEANSE

For those of you who prefer a more prescriptive program, here is a list of juices we've developed based on the recipes at the end of the book that can be used for your Cleanse. Or you can drink the same juices each day...that's perfectly fine! You'll see that the juice recipes section in the back of the book instructs you to mix and match juices as you like, as long as you have a certain number of fruit juice and vegetable juices on each day, depending on your level.

Level 1
DAY ONE
1. Greens with Apple
2. Grapefruit-Strawberry-Mint
3. Cherry-Banana-Peach
4. Pineapple-Raspberry-Mint
5. Spinach-Blueberry-Apple-Lemon
6. Raw Chocolate Milk

DAY TWO
1. Greens with Apple
2. Grapefruit-Strawberry-Mint
3. Grape-Cucumber-Pear
4. Spinach-Blueberry-Apple-Lemon
5. Strawberry-Apple-Beet
6. Easy Cashew Milk

DAY THREE
1. Greens with Apple
2. Spinach-Blueberry-Apple-Lemon
3. Pineapple-Raspberry-Mint
4. Cherry-Banana-Peach
5. Grape-Cucumber-Pear
6. Raw Chocolate Milk

Level 2
DAY ONE
1. Greens with Apple
2. Pineapple-Mint

3. Spinach-Blueberry-Apple-Lemon
4. Watermelon
5. Greens with Apple
6. Easy Cashew Milk

DAY TWO
1. Greens with Apple
2. Pineapple-Mint
3. Greens with Apple/Ginger
4. Watermelon
5. Greens with Apple
6. Easy Cashew Milk

DAY THREE
1. Greens with Apple
2. Pineapple-Mint
3. Spinach-Blueberry-Apple-Lemon
4. Watermelon
5. Greens with Apple
6. Easy Cashew Milk

Level 3
DAY ONE
1. Greens with Apple
2. Greens with Apple
3. Greens with Apple
4. Grape-Cucumber-Pear
5. Greens with Apple/Ginger
6. Easy Cashew Milk

DAY TWO
1. Greens with Apple
2. Grape-Cucumber-Pear

3. Greens with Apple
4. Greens with Apple/Ginger
5. Greens with Apple
6. Easy Cashew Milk

DAY THREE
1. Greens with Apple
2. Grape-Cucumber-Pear
3. Greens with Apple
4. Greens with Apple/Ginger
5. Greens with Apple
6. Easy Cashew Milk

Comparing the Levels

The main differences among the three levels have to do with sugar content and experience—that is, how ready your system is to take on the challenge of raw juice. This is based on what your diet is like to begin with, and how intensely you prepare for the Cleanse (more on preparation in the next chapter). Renovation has the most calories, followed by Foundation and Excavation. So you're less likely to get hungry on the Renovation Cleanse.

Renovator also contains the most sugar (all-natural from the fruit and agave nectar). This is particularly important for people who have never done a Cleanse before and/or never tasted a green juice—as noted before, Level 1 juices are simply easier to take because they're sweeter, with more fruit than either of the other two levels.

We also want to say a few words about the difference between the fruit juices and the green juices. While both are important for detoxification and optimal nutrition, the green juice has a strong alkalizing effect while the fruit juices are more acidic and, thus, more astringent. We like to think of the fruit juices as "digging up" the gunk, and the green juice "moving it out."

So which level are you? We try to leave that up to you, our client. Because as we said earlier, the level you are today is not necessarily the level you will be next month. Having said that, we think that the following quiz should be helpful in guiding you toward the best level for you now.

THE 3-DAY CLEANSE DETOX QUIZ

Rate each symptom on a scale of 0 to 4 as follows:

0. I never experience this.
1. I experience this less than once a month.
2. I experience this at least once a month.
3. I experience this no more than once or twice a week on average.
4. I experience this most days.

	0	1	2	3	4
DIGESTIVE SYSTEM					
Bloated feeling					
Constipation					
Diarrhea					
Gas					
Heartburn/acid reflux					
Nausea/vomiting					
RESPIRATORY SYSTEM					
Allergies					
Asthma/wheezing					
Congestion					
Cough					
Postnasal drip					
Sinusitis					

	0	1	2	3	4
JOINT/MUSCLES					
Backache					
Feeling of weakness					
Joint pain					
Neck/shoulder pain					
Stiffness/limited movement					
HEAD/MEMORY					
Difficulty making decisions					
Dizziness					
Faintness					
Headache					
Inability to concentrate					
Poor memory/forgetting things					
Pressure behind the eyes					
SKIN/HAIR/NAILS					
Acne					
Brittle nails					
Blotchy skin					
Dandruff					
Dry skin					
Hair loss					
Hives					
Oily skin					
EMOTIONAL HEALTH					
Angry					
Anxious					
Depressed					

	0	1	2	3	4
Mood swings					
Nervous					
Sad					
ENERGY/ACTIVITY					
Difficulty waking up in the morning					
Insomnia					
Lack of energy/sluggish feeling					
Tired/fatigued					
MOUTH/THROAT					
Canker sores					
Chapped lips					
Dry mouth					
Sore throat					
EYES					
Blurred vision					
Dark circles					
Itchy/watery eyes					
Puffy eyelids					
Red eyes					
APPETITE					
Binge eating/drinking					
Cravings					
Difficulty losing weight					
Drink alcohol					
TOTAL POSSIBLE: 220					

Now complete the following questions about your lifestyle.
0. Never
1. Occasionally
2. At least once a month
3. At least once a week
4. Most days

How often do you...
1. Exercise for 30 minutes or more?
2. Have sex?
3. Fast?
4. Drink alcohol?
5. Eat red meat?
6. Get at least five servings of fruit or vegetables?
7. Eat in front of the TV or computer?
8. Nap?
9. Do something relaxing just for yourself?
10. Use chemicals around your house or yard (i.e., bleach, ammonia, weed spray, bug killer, etc.)?
11. Drink filtered water?

To get your score:
[total score from section 1] + [total score from section 2, questions 1, 2, 3, 6, 8, 9, and 11] – [total score from questions 4, 5, 7, and 10]

What is your total score?
    0–10. Get out of here! You're doing so well we're not even sure you *need* the Cleanse! Still, a Level 1 Cleanse (Renovation) never hurt anyone!
    11–20. You're doing okay, but it's good that you're doing the Cleanse. Consider Level 1 (Renovation) or 2 (Foundation).
    21–35. You are teetering on the edge of the red (danger)

zone. You should consider the Level 2 (Foundation) or Level 3 (Excavation) Cleanse.

35+. You know you're in trouble. You will need a Level 3 (Excavation) Cleanse, but should begin with a Level 1 Cleanse to ease into it.

Cleanse Clients Ask...
What if I have Candida or don't want so much sugar?
Candida albicans is a fungus that lives on about 80 percent of all people. If you have a healthy immune system and a healthy diet, the two of you coexist quite comfortably. But if your immune system weakens, you take antibiotics (which kills off "good" bacteria that can keep the fungus in check), or you follow a high-sugar diet (which feeds the fungus), Candida can grow out of control. The result could be as relatively benign as a yeast infection, or as serious as candidiasis, a systemic disease that can land you in the hospital.

Since a high-sugar diet feeds Candida, people who are susceptible to the fungal overgrowth often try to limit their intake of sugar, whether natural or added. If you want to limit your sugar intake, we recommend the Excavation Level of the Cleanse (Level 3), since it has the lowest sugar content of all the Cleanses.

GET TO KNOW THE JUICES

Because the juices are the essence of the ingredients from which they are made, the purity of those ingredients is critical. We already talked about the importance of organic produce, preferably purchased from a farmer's market or local farm. During the spring, summer, and fall, you might even be able to use produce out of your garden! Unless you are using produce from your own organic garden, we still want you to clean the fruits and vegetables *very* well.

Now let's talk about *why* these specific ingredients were chosen for our juices, and how they can help with detoxing and healing. We call this our "Magic Ingredients List."

Agave. You may know this plant primarily for its contribution to your favorite mixer, tequila. But it also has medicinal uses. Teas made from the leaves have traditionally been drunk to relieve constipation and gas, as a diuretic, and to soothe the pain of arthritis. We use the nectar as a natural sweetener for our juices.

Apples. Apples contain two important types of fiber: insoluble fiber, found in the skin, and soluble fiber (pectin), found in the flesh (you'll notice we don't peel our apples before throwing them into the juicer). Fiber is important to any healthy diet since it fills you up without filling you out. It does that because our bodies can't digest fiber. Instead, the fiber also binds toxins in the gut and escorts them out of you via . . . well, you know.

In the long term, fiber works wonders at keeping cholesterol levels low, with some studies suggesting that just an apple a day (yeah, we know!) can help maintain a healthy cholesterol level. That's because fiber binds to bile acids in the gut, forcing the liver to make more bile. To do that, the liver has to break down cholesterol!

Like all fruits and vegetables, apples are antioxidant powerhouses. This means they can work better at preventing or improving disease than many medications. For instance, one study found that as little as two apples a day could reduce your risk of asthma by nearly a third!

Apples are also alkalizing, meaning they are important to maintaining a balanced pH in your blood during the Cleanse.

Bananas. The banana's best benefit lies in its potassium. Eat enough foods high in potassium and you can slash your risk of heart attack and high blood pressure, not to mention leg cramps. Bananas can also help soothe acidy stomachs.

Blueberries. When it comes to antioxidants, dark berries such as blueberries and blackberries top the scale. They're also good sources of quercetin, a phytochemical (plant-based compound) that helps protect against infectious diseases such as the flu, and of compounds that repair free radical damage in the eyes, preventing age-related macular degeneration.

Beets. One of the commercial juices we make, and several of the recipes and juices we provide, call for beets. We know beets aren't everyone's cup of tea, but they're terrific sources of a powerful antioxidant called betacyanin, which helps protect against the kind of DNA damage that can lead to cancer. Beets are also awesome sources of iron, terrific for those of you who are cutting back on or cutting out meat and shellfish.

Carrots. Carrots and other deep orange and yellow vegetables are rich in carotenoids, phytochemicals that help reduce the risk of heart disease, among other health benefits. They are also rich in lutein, a phytochemical shown to prevent macular degeneration, and beta-carotene, a terrific antioxidant that helps strengthen the immune system. Other studies find that the varied phytochemicals in carrots also help protect against numerous cancers.

Cashews. Many of our clients tell us that our cashew nut milk is their favorite. They liken it to dessert, say it fills them up more than the other juices, and rave about its "mouth feel." We're glad they like the taste, but we're primarily thrilled with the nutritional benefits of the cashews. Cashews are rich sources of zinc, an essential mineral used to build collagen, an essential element in healthy, young-looking skin and nails. Cashews also contain arginine, which acts to dilate blood vessels in much the same way as nitroglycerine. One other benefit we'd like to highlight: high levels of vitamin E, one of the most potent food-based antioxidants.

Cayenne. Compounds in peppers such as cayenne have a variety of benefits, including anticancer properties. One compound, capsaicin, is often used as a topical pain reliever for conditions such as arthritis and neuropathic pain. Peppers are also fantastic decongestants. Remember the last time you ate a really spicy food? You probably felt your sinuses clear almost immediately. That's why cayenne is such an important ingredient in our juices.

Celery. Celery is a vital part of the "greens" part of any juice containing greens, whether you make it on your own or purchase it from us. Celery, celery root, and celery seed are included in several of our recipes and juices for a variety of reasons. First, celery is a natural diuretic. Second, celery is one of the best sources of phthalides, phytonutrients with significant blood pressure–lowering benefits. They also help quell inflammation. Even more important when it comes to the Cleanse, phthalides also stimulate the production of an enzyme called glutathione S-transferase (GST), which plays a major role in detoxification.

Cinnamon. Cinnamon is what gives our cashew milk its wonderful flavor. But cinnamon does far more than just spice up pumpkin pies! It also helps stabilize and control blood sugar by increasing insulin sensitivity, even in people with diabetes. Cinnamon is also known as a "carminative," a plant that helps relieve gas and bloating. There's also some evidence that it can help prevent or improve yeast infections such as candidiasis.

Cucumber. Cucumbers, like celery, are found in all "greens" juices. Cucumbers are valuable not just for their water content (they're 95% water), but also because they contain ascorbic acid and caffeic acid, natural diuretics. So cucumbers serve an important diuretic function in the Cleanse, stimulating the kidneys and helping flush away toxins (this is why lying down with a couple of cucumber slices over your eyes relieves puffiness). Cucumbers' high fiber content (found in the skin and seeds) also helps clean out your colon, which is why a couple of cucumbers

a day are often recommended for people suffering from constipation. Because cucumbers are so alkaline, they are also helpful
at reducing acids, and are often recommended for people with
heartburn or "acid stomach." In fact, they can actually work
faster than an antacid at soothing that burning feeling.

Cucumbers are also high in the mineral silica, needed for
strong nails, bones, tendons, and muscles, as well as potassium
and magnesium. They also contain fluorine, a trace element you
probably know best as fluoride. Fluorine is essential for preventing cavities and building strong bone.

Cherries. Cherries' anti-inflammatory properties are the reason they have traditionally been used as a "cure" for gout and
arthritis, painful conditions related to inflammation. They are
also one of the few foods that contain the antioxidant vitamin
E. Studies find that high levels of vitamin E from food can help
prevent heart disease.

Cilantro. Long known as a key ingredient in salsa and other
Mexican dishes, cilantro, or coriander, as its seeds are called, is
rich in phytonutrients that have antibiotic properties. Cilantro
has also been shown to reduce cholesterol and inflammation.

Ginger. Ginger is a natural anti-inflammatory, with studies
showing extracts can help relieve the pain of arthritis and labo-
ratory research suggesting its anti-inflammatory effects may protect against heart disease, cancer, and Alzheimer's disease. Other
benefits include its ability to reduce cholesterol, stem nausea and
motion sickness, and reduce the risk of blood clots.

Grapefruit. We incorporated grapefruit into the 3-Day
Cleanse because it contains so many important antioxidants.
There's vitamin C, of course, but also lycopene, limonoids (also
found in lemons and limes), and naringin. All you need to know
is that their health benefits seem to go on and on, with studies
finding that grapefruit compounds can protect against numerous
cancers, reduce the risk of kidney stones, and lower cholesterol,
among other benefits.

Grapes. Grapes are perhaps best known as a primary source of the antioxidant resveratrol, which some studies suggest may help with weight loss and extend the lifespan. It also attacks damaging free radicals.

Kale. Kale is one of those dark, leafy greens that pack a nutritional powerhouse in every bite. It is an excellent source of bone-building calcium and magnesium, and also a terrific place to get the antioxidant quercetin, a flavonoid with immune-strengthening benefits thanks to its ability to prevent viruses from multiplying.

Lemons and limes. Wondering why we recommend you start your Cleanse with a cup of hot water and lemon juice? Because the acidity in lemon helps counter the alkaline nature of your blood that remains after a night without food, rebalancing your blood's pH. (Plus, the warm water with the acidic flavoring is a wonderful way to gently wake up your digestive system and get things, uh, moving.) The same goes for limes. Both are also rich in vitamin C, a powerful antioxidant that also helps strengthen the immune system. Last but certainly not least, the flavonoid compounds in lemons and limes, particularly limonin, have powerful anticancer and cholesterol-lowering benefits.

Mint. We add mint to several Cleanse juices both for its bold flavoring and for its strong anti-inflammatory benefits. Mint also fights bacteria, including the nasty bugs in your mouth that cause cavities and gum disease.

Parsley. Parsley is actually an herb, one that does far more than just decorate a dinner plate. It is a digestif, meaning it freshens your breath and help prevent post-meal heartburn; it's a great source of vitamin K, important for healthy bone and blood clotting; and it contains compounds shown to inhibit cancer and lower cholesterol. It is also a natural diuretic and a great source of vitamin C.

Peaches. As with all fruits, peaches provide natural sweetness to our juices. But they are also rich sources of zeaxanthin and lutein, compounds found in food that we need to protect our eyes from age-related macular degeneration.

Pineapple. Pineapple is a natural source of bromelain, an enzyme with significant anti-inflammatory properties. It is used in some countries to speed healing after surgery. Bromelain also helps with digestion, particularly of protein. This tropical fruit is also a good source of manganese, a mineral important to healthy bone, skin, nails and cartilage, and of vitamin C.

Raspberries. These dark red berries are rich in anthocyanins, flavonoids with powerful anticancer properties. Raspberries also have strong antifungal properties and are packed with manganese, a trace mineral vital for energy production and breaking down fat and cholesterol.

Romaine lettuce. Romaine lettuce is also an essential ingredient in our "green" juices. Romaine and other dark green lettuces are one of your best dietary sources of vitamin K, a natural blood thinner and diuretic. That's why we add romaine: to assist with kidney and blood detoxification. Packed with vitamin C and beta-carotene, romaine is also a powerful antioxidant, *protecting* the liver, kidneys, and other detoxifying organs during your Cleanse.

Spinach. Another powerful part of our "green" juices, every forkful (or sip) of spinach is like getting a handful of vitamins and minerals. Spinach is filled with phytonutrients critical for healthy vision. It is also one of our best dietary sources of the powerful antioxidant vitamin E, which can stimulate the immune system and keep brain cells (aka your memory) healthy with its ability to slurp up damaging free radicals. And of course, let's not forget the high iron content of spinach, essential for adequate hemoglobin production, which is, after all, a major component of energy. Spinach is also one of the best sources of chlorophyll, which contains magnesium, helpful for reducing the acidity of your blood.

Strawberries. We consider strawberries a power food, with just one cup providing more than an entire day's worth of vitamin C.

Strawberries are also one of the best sources of ellagic acid, which has major anticancer properties.

Watermelon. We love watermelon not just for its sweet taste, but for its powerful antioxidant and anti-inflammatory properties. It is a fabulous source of vitamin C and beta-carotene, and a great source of lycopene, shown to help prevent vision-related problems.

Choose Your Herbs Wisely	
To...	**Chew on or brew into a tea**
Expel gas	Aniseed, parsley, dill, ginger, fennel
Stimulate digestion	Cinnamon, spearmint, ginger, cloves, nutmeg, burdock, licorice, peppermint
Soothe irritation	Flax, marshmallow root, fenugreek
Relieve constipation	Dandelion root, cascara bark, barberry bark, rhubarb

TIME TO MOVE ON

Now that you know what level Cleanse you're going to start with and why our juices are so nutritious and healthy, it's time to begin the real work—preparing for the Cleanse. Don't worry...we cover it all in the next chapter.

CHAPTER 4

Preparing to Cleanse

I prefer to ease into my Cleanses, getting off sugar and caffeine (though I no longer drink coffee at all) and packaged foods for about three days leading up to the juice fasting. However, the very first time I tried the Cleanse, I didn't prepare at all. I got very nauseous and headachey the first day! That was enough to teach me to prepare in advance!

—Peggy

Yes! We know! You're excited to get started. You want to begin drinking, begin flushing, get that incredibly clean, healthy feeling as your body detoxes. And we're excited *for* you!

But listen up. You wouldn't run in a marathon without preparing first, would you?

Right. Well, the same holds true for the 3-Day Cleanse.

If you don't prepare properly for the Cleanse, you will feel hungrier and have more detox symptoms such as headaches, bloating, irritability, and nausea, which occur from a digestive system that was zooming along at 60 miles per hour and just had the brakes slammed on. You have to apply the brake gently and slowly. You have to "train" your digestive system for the Cleanse by gradually transitioning from your dense diet, which puts your digestive system into heavy work mode, to the lighter state it will find itself in during the Cleanse.

Here's what *not* to do...

I didn't prepare at all the first time. In fact, my boyfriend and I ordered our favorite pizza from Chicago via FedEx (yes, FedEx—see the problem!!??) and ate it the night before.

No, we did *not* make that up! This came from Suzy. She knew the pizza thing was not such a good idea, but as she noted, "I'm an all-or-nothing person. So it's hard for me to turn off one little thing at a time...or wind down." Instead, she said, she prepares for her Cleanses by saying, "Okay the party's over, I'm giving up everything just for a short time to see how it goes." Unfortunately, then, she doesn't do the things we recommend (all pulled together in one neat list beginning just below), and thus, she suffers.

Some of you may decide to order your juices instead of making them. If you do, you might find you're hungry while you're waiting for your delivery. Feel free to grab a piece of fruit in that case.

Remember, don't torture yourself! This is supposed to be fun and freeing, not awful. Also, if you make your own juices, have all the produce for the first day already washed and ready to go first thing in the morning.

PREPARING FOR THE CLEANSE

Okay, so what do we mean when we say "prepare"? Here are our top tips:

1. **Wean yourself off coffee and other caffeinated drinks a week before you plan to start the Cleanse.** This will help prevent a caffeine-withdrawal headache. The easiest way to do this is slowly. The first day, go with a 1:2 ratio: one-third decaf, two-thirds caffeine. The next day, make it 50-50. Then mostly decaf with a little caffeine. Day 4, you should be decaf only. Day 5, drink only a half-cup of decaf (which, contrary to its name, still contains *some* caffeine). On Day 6, the day before your Cleanse begins, you should be able to go all day without caffeine and without a headache. And don't forget the other sources of caffeine in your diet: soft drinks, chocolate, and painkillers such as Excedrin.

   Now, we know that many of you have the "I must have hot liquid down my throat before I can open my eyes" syndrome.

No worries. Start your day with a cup of herbal tea or hot water and lemon. And if you simply can't get past the caffeine thing, we suggest green tea. Yes, it has caffeine, but it contains far less than coffee plus it's a fabulous source of those all-important antitoxin antioxidants.

2. **Cut out the salt.** After all, you'll be cutting out the salt on the Cleanse. None of our juices have even one grain of added salt. But did you know that many vegetables on their own have a lot of sodium? Celery is one, which is why it's such a good diuretic. If you cut back on salt *now,* the salt-free diet of the Cleanse won't be such a shock to your system. The best way to reduce your sodium intake is to do two things: Stop eating processed foods, which are loaded with sodium, and stop eating fast food. 'Nuff said.

3. **Skip the sugar.** You will be shocked, yes, absolutely shocked, to learn just how sweet our juices are *without any added sugar.* To get the full impact of this sweetness, we want you to cut out all foods that contain added sweeteners in the day or two before your Cleanse. That means all "natural" and artificial sweeteners (and for the record, honey, molasses, and natural cane sugar are all just as bad as "table" sugar when it comes to added sugar). It also means nixing the candy, cake, cookies, and believe it or not, most processed foods, which are typically loaded up with sugar. Which brings us to our next recommendation.

4. **Pretend you're a vegetarian.** Or at least go meatless for a couple of days. Trust us...a steak and martini the night before your Cleanse is so *not* the way to go! (Neither is Fed-Exing yourself a pizza, but we've already covered that topic.) Fish is okay. Just make sure that the largest portion of all your meals for two days before the Cleanse comes from fruit and/or vegetables. Which brings us to one of the most important pre-Cleanse steps: load up on fruits and vegetables. After all, that's what you'll be consuming over the next few days, so get

your system used to it. It's really not that complicated. Here are five ways to "sneak" in extra veggies and fruit:

- **Start the morning with a smoothie.** You'll find several superdelicious recipes beginning on page 207. If you need extra protein, add a couple of tablespoons of almond or cashew butter (organic, unsweetened, and unsalted, please). Skip the peanut butter; peanuts are often difficult to digest.
- **Snack on the stuff.** If you're too lazy...uh, *busy* to cut up fresh veggies every time you want a snack, pick up a veggie tray at the supermarket. Same goes for fruit. Most supermarkets these days offer fruits and veggies that are presliced, peeled, and ready for your mouth or the microwave. And how about grapes or a banana? The ultimate convenience foods!

  Here's a tip: Keep the fruit out on the counter. It's so much easier to grab an apple from a bowl on the counter than it is to *ooopppenn* the refrigerator...lean in...puuuulll out the drawer...and choose the apple. Plus, it's usually too cold and then it hurts your teeth!
- **Serve up a super salad.** Instead of a sandwich for lunch, make yours a super salad. Start with a bag (or two) of organic lettuce and add a whole diced red pepper, a handful of grape tomatoes, cucumbers, avocados, and any other fresh-cut veggies you can find. There's no limit to how many vegetables you can put into a salad. See the recipe section for more ideas.
- **Sneak in the veggies.** Plan on pasta for dinner. Then make a tomato sauce with fresh or canned tomatoes. But don't stop there. The onions and garlic you brown for the sauce count as veggies. Now finely dice or shred several carrots, a couple of peppers, and some yellow squash or zucchini. Got kids (or a husband) who won't eat chunky spaghetti

sauce? No worries. Just puree the veggies and mix them into the sauce. They'll never know! If you really want to up the veggies in your life, serve the sauce over shredded spaghetti squash instead of pasta.

- **Serve soup.** Vegetable soup, of course. But do us a favor and make it yourself. Yes, we're serious. No, it's not complicated! In fact, we have more than half a dozen soup recipes beginning on page 141 that even someone who only passes through the kitchen to get to the den could manage. And if all else fails and you must turn to the canned stuff, by all means get the organic, low-salt, no-sugar soup. Please?

5. **Up your liquid volume.** No, in this case we're not talking about a good bottle of Oregon Pinot Noir. We're talking about water. Lots and lots of water. And make sure it's filtered (if you don't remember why, review the information on toxic water on page 19). The extra fluid will help you start your Cleanse early. We suggest you buy a 24-ounce refillable bottle and, starting in the morning, make sure you empty and refill it (via drinking) at least four times a day. Not crazy about plain water? Squeeze a lemon or lime into it. Just keep drinking (and peeing). If your urine is nearly as pale as water, you're doing great.

6. **Cut out the dairy.** That means milk, ice cream, cheese, yogurt, butter...anything that comes from a cow, goat, or sheep. Simply put, there is no place for dairy in a raw food/juice program. That's because a big part of our Cleanse philosophy is that you should incorporate more fresh, "live" foods into your diet and eliminate processed and difficult-to-digest items such as meat and dairy. This doesn't have to be a permanent change (although you'll feel much better overall if it is), but it does need to be a key component of the pre-, during-, and post-Cleanse time frame. Plus, as you probably know, many of us are lactose intolerant, meaning we can't digest the sugar

in dairy. This leads to all sorts of unpleasant intestinal issues such as constipation and gas. Keep away from soy milk since is a highly acidic food. It is also highly processed, and can increase levels of mucus in your intestines.

7. **Eat gingerly the day before.** See Steps 1 through 6 for the specifics. Why? If you don't prepare properly, it's not necessarily that disaster will bring you to your knees. It's a matter of how you will feel. If you eat a particularly dense meal the night before you begin your Cleanse—think meat (even fish) and heavy starches like French fries—your body will be in heavy digestion mode the following day, ready to tackle another dense meal. So when it encounters the light, simple, raw juice instead, you may end up feeling woozy, nauseated, and extremely hungry because your body has been in work mode for so long. Those digestive juices are still churning, but now they have nothing to break down.

To prep for the Cleanse, I reduced my caloric intake the day before by eating fruit and fresh fruit juice. It helped me to become accustomed to the Cleanse and ease into the program.

—RACHEL

To make it even easier for you to prepare for the Cleanse, we've prepared the following three-day menu for you leading up to the Cleanse itself. All the recipes can found beginning on page 135. Remember, the focus is on gradually transitioning from "denser" foods that require more digestion to lighter foods that will "exit" your system quicker.

If you're into making your own juices, we *always* recommend a green juice for breakfast. This is simply the best bet to "break your fast" no matter where you are in the Cleanse cycle because your body will absorb it quickest and easiest, preparing your system for the rest of the day.

Three Days Pre-Cleanse

Breakfast: Smoothie of your choice or two bananas.

Lunch: Lentil Salad (recipe on page 160).

Snack: Lärabar. These energy bars are made with unsweetened fruits, nuts, and spices, with each type containing no more than six ingredients, all natural, all raw. They are also gluten, soy, and dairy free; vegan; and kosher. They come in a variety of flavors. You can find them in specialty and health food stores, or online at www.larabar.com.

Dinner: Sea Vegetable Salad with Ginger-Miso Dressing (recipe page 156) and Asian Cold Noodles with Spicy Almond Dressing (recipe page 179).

Two Days Pre-Cleanse

Breakfast: Fresh fruit, one piece at a time, preferably "watery" fruits such as plums, peaches, and apples. Just one type, however. You can eat as much as you want until you feel satisfied, but not completely full. Remember, it takes about twenty minutes for your brain to receive a message from your stomach that you're full. If you keep eating without allowing that message time to come through, you will feel overfull and sick.

Lunch: Veggie Tacos with Guacamole (recipes pages 185 and 195). Sprouted corn tortillas are typically found in the freezer section of a good health food store. Their chewy texture and nutty flavor are absolutely amazing! We provide two recipes for Guacamole on page 195; choose whichever you prefer. Just remember: No cheese!

Snack: Spicy Edamame Hummus (recipe page 196) with cut veggies.

Dinner: Greenmarket Salad (recipe page 154) with Basic Vinaigrette (recipe page 166) and Steamed Artichoke with Lemon Aioli (recipe page 191).

One Day Pre-Cleanse

Breakfast: Watermelon or papaya, as much as you want.
Lunch: Gazpacho (recipe page 142).
Snack: Fresh fruit, one to two pieces.
Dinner: Shaved Fennel Salad (recipe page 157).

Cleanse!

Cleanse Clients Ask...
Can I smoke on the Cleanse?

Surely you already know the answer to this! In case
you don't, here it is...*no!* The whole point of the
Cleanse is to detox, not to add *more* toxins through
smoking. The same goes for drinking alcohol.
Both add toxins to your system and stress the very
detoxification organs you're trying to rest.

Also consider this...preparing for the Cleanse is an
ideal time to quit smoking (or drinking). Not only will
you be doing some deep detoxing, clearing out years
of cigarette-related toxins, but the Cleanse itself could
help you stay smoke-free. After all, if you just spent
days clearing out the toxins in your body, why would
you want to undo all that work with just a single
cigarette? In fact, some of our clients do the Cleanse as
a part of quitting smoking.

As Kathy wrote us: "I am a small person to start
with, at 5'6" and 115 pounds (well, I'm 113 now),
and I didn't cleanse to lose weight. I had just made
the decision to stop smoking—finally—and the
Cleanse seemed like a logical way to rid my body of
the nicotine and allow myself a much better chance of
success. Well, I have to share that the Cleanse really

did allow me to not crave cigarettes much at all. Now that I have 3 days under my belt and no withdrawal symptoms, I'm confident this time I will succeed. In addition to all of the other benefits of the Cleanse, if there is anyone who wants to quit smoking—this is surely the way to begin."

Studies find that it takes, on average, twenty-one days to break a habit (or form a habit). So our suggestion, if you're up for it, is that you undertake a 21-Day Cleanse combined with raw food recipes from the selection beginning on page 135. By the end of the Cleanse, you should be over your smoking (alcohol, nail biting, hair pulling, etc.) habit for good.

MAKING YOUR OWN JUICES

To make the juices listed in the previous chapter, you need a juicer. Sure, you could throw everything into the blender; but that results in a high-pulp product. The more pulp in a juice, the more energy your body has to spend on digestion. This slows the detox process. Conversely, the less pulp in the blend, the less your digestive system has to work, speeding up and deepening the detox.

There are hundreds of juicer models on the market. Here is what you need to know about juicers, along with our personal recommendations.

At BluePrintCleanse, we use a commercial hydraulic press to extract the juices from the fruits, vegetables, herbs, spices, and nuts in our packaged juices. Hydraulic presses use a dual twin-gear system to literally squeeze items between two rollers, extracting so much juice that the resulting pulp is nearly dry. Comparisons between various juicers show that this approach extracts three to five times more juice (and, thus, three to five times more vitamins and minerals) than other juicers.

Creating the juice is a two-part process. First, we cut and grind the ingredients, then we put them into the press. Because the press moves relatively slowly, little oxygen gets into the juice, preventing oxidation and ensuring it stays fresh for up to three days.

In addition to hydraulic juicers, the other main types of juicers are masticating and centrifugal. The pros and cons of each, along with our recommendations, are outlined below.

Questions to Ask Before Purchasing a Juicer

- **What will I use it for?** Some juicers are best for fruits, which are easy to break down, others for vegetables, which are more fibrous. Centrifugal juicers and some masticating juicers, for instance, aren't great with leafy greens and wheatgrass.
- **How often will I use it?** You want a juicer that can stand up to heavy use if you plan to use it often; but if you're just interested in a few glasses a month, no need to spend a huge amount.
- **How loud can I stand it?** Some juicers are quieter than others.
- **How fast should it be?** Centrifugal juicers, for instance, are the fastest.
- **How much can I spend?** Juicers range from about a hundred to thousands of dollars. Expect to spend a couple hundred for a decent home juicer.
- **How long do I want the warranty?** Longer warranties may cost more.

Masticating juicers. These juicers use a single gear to "chew" fiber and break down cell walls. It takes longer, but produces a better juice. Our favorite is the Plastaket Champion Juicer, which, its manufacturer claims, "provides more fiber, enzymes, vitamins and trace minerals... resulting in the darker, richer color of the juice and a sweeter, richer more full-bodied flavor." We also like this type of juicer for its ability to homogenize, or emulsify, varied ingredients, ensuring that even nut butters and sauces stay mixed and don't separate out into their individual ingredients. Masticating juicers also use less heat and introduce less air into the juice, so juices stay fresh longer. The Champion Juicer is also super easy to clean. It retails for around $235.

Centrifugal juicers. These juicers use centrifugal force to extract juice from ground fruit and vegetables in much the same way your washing machine extracts water while on the spin cycle. The juicers typically have two cycles; one grinds the fruit and veggies, the other spins it, pushing the pulp to the back of the machine, where it is ejected. This is one of the fastest ways to juice.

However, these juicers leave a fair amount of pulp in the juice. You also need to drink the juice right away because the process introduces a lot of air into the juice, leading to oxidation (you'll know a juice has oxidized when it turns brown—the same process is at work when you leave a cut apple or pear exposed to the air). These juicers are great with fruits, pretty good with greens, but can't be used with wheatgrass. They're best if you're making small amounts of juice. We recommend the Omega 1000 and 4000 (about $200) and the Breville Juice Fountain Elite, a sleek, functional, and easy-to-use machine that retails for about $500.

Hydraulic (triturating) juicers. Hydraulic juicers are generally the most expensive and labor intensive of all the juicers. But this is the type we use, and the type we recommend for people who plan to make juices and the 3-Day Cleanse a regular part of their lives. Hydraulic juicers run at slower speeds, so less air is incorporated into the juice. Thus, your juice stays fresher longer and can be refrigerated for a few days. Hydraulic juicers can be used with every type of fruit, vegetable, nut, etc., even wheatgrass. Like masticating juicers, they also homogenize ingredients, making them ideal for items that might otherwise separate. Plus, since this type of juicer eliminates nearly all the pulp, the juice is much easier to assimilate into your system. Our favorite for home juicers is the Norwalk Hydraulic Press, which retails for about $2,000.

OTHER JUICERS

In addition to the "do nearly everything" juicers, you can buy juicers designed just for citrus fruits (citrus presses) or wheatgrass (wheatgrass juicers). The citrus presses eliminate the need to peel an orange, grapefruit, lemon, or lime (which you typically need to do before juicing because the rind can be so bitter). Instead, you just slice the fruit in half and put the cut side down on the juice press. Our favorite here is the Breville Citrus Juice Press, which retails for about $190. Our choice for wheatgrass juicers is the Lexen Healthyjuicer, about $50.

Tips for Home Juicing

1. The juices you make at home are not pasteurized, so they should be drunk immediately. If you let them sit, the enzymes will lose their vibrancy. The juices we make commercially stay fresh for three days because of the press process, but anything made with a centrifugal juicer has too much pulp to stay fresh for an extended time.

2. A brown juice is an oxidized juice. Toss it.

3. Use organic fruits and vegetables if possible. If not, make sure you clean the produce very well with either an electric produce cleaner or a produce cleaning solution.

4. Peel citrus fruits, kiwis, papayas, and pineapple before juicing. Other produce can be juiced with the peel intact. In fact, we recommend it; the peels of many fruits and vegetables are great sources of fiber and nutrients. When juicing citrus fruits in a regular juicer, leave the fine white "pith," a source of valuable nutrients.

5. To reduce strain on your juicer, slice or cut the produce before juicing.

Other Kitchen Gadgets

The following will make preparing the recipes that begin on page 135 ever so much easier!

Immersion blender. It's a big help to have a handheld device when making blended soups, since pouring hot liquid from pot to blender and back can be messy. That's why we love our Cuisinart Smart Stick Hand Blender (i.e., immersion blender). It retails for about $30. It's not cordless, but we don't think a cordless immersion blender is required, since who doesn't have a stove with a nearby outlet?

Mandoline/box slicer. We couldn't live without this gadget. It's fabulous for making shaved vegetable salads, as well as for cucumbers, fennel (ideal!), radishes, carrots, and onions. We recommend the Benriner/Asian mandoline, about $50.

Microplane grater. Simply the best for grating fresh ginger and hard cheeses like Parmesan and for zesting citrus fruits. You can pick up one at any big box store for a few dollars.

Minichopper/food processer. This gadget is absolutely critical. You don't want to have to clean out a big blender every time you prepare a salad. It is also ideal for salad dressings and dips. Our favorite (don't laugh) is the as-seen-on-TV Magic Bullet. We probably use ours at least four times a week, and it's super easy to clean, even without a dish-washer. You can find it online for about $50.

CHAPTER 5

The Cleanse!

I found that it was pretty essential to have a buddy, as I was on the verge of cheating right from the start. By the end of day one, I was ready to stuff my face with a cheeseburger. One of the hardest parts of the day was when my friend and I went to a fancy party where everyone was sipping champagne. Had she not been there to keep me on track, I would have probably caved and had a glass.

—SHERRIL

In this chapter, we walk you through a typical 3-Day Cleanse, the one most of our clients choose. We provide plenty of stories from clients so you can hear firsthand about real people's real experiences. You'll quickly see how different everyone's experiences are and, we hope, realize that there is no "typical" Cleanse.

On page 98 we provide a list of questions we often get (along with the answers) to guide you in your Cleanse. And on page 109 we provide a chart showing which symptoms are "normal" and which are not...along with advice to make your Cleanse easier.

DAY 1

The first morning of your Cleanse should begin with water or, even better, water with lemon. Hot is best because it gets your bowels moving, waking up your system. From there, start your morning with a green juice. The green juice is the gentlest way to get your digestive system working after a night of fasting. After that, drink either a green or a fruit juice throughout the day, at least one hour apart.

Also drink at least 12 ounces of water, green tea (regular or decaf), and/or herbal tea, as much as you like, to flush out your system and help eliminate the toxins. Oh, a word about tea: We are often asked about drinking kombucha tea while on the Cleanse. While it's an excellent drink for digestion because it's loaded with probiotics (more on probiotics on page 108), it also contains processed sugar and black tea, neither of which we recommend during your Cleanse. The added sugar will put more strain on your digestion and send your blood sugar soaring and then crashing, and the black tea is loaded with caffeine. Save the kombucha for a post-Cleanse treat.

Drink the nut milk at least two hours before bed. We recommend this for two reasons. One, the nut milk has the most fat and protein so it will keep you full longer, throughout the night, so you don't wake up starving. We ask you to drink it at least two hours before you go to sleep because eating or drinking closer to bedtime can interfere with your sleep and doesn't give your digestive system enough of a rest. However... we do have clients who need a little something extra first thing in the morning. So if you must, have a quarter or a half of the nut milk along with your green juice.

You may find that in the morning you're very hungry and drink two juices within two hours. That's fine. Then you may find that you're not hungry for five hours and so don't drink anything. That's fine, too. Don't be surprised to find that as the day goes on, you feel *less* hungry.

Cleanse Clients Ask...
Can I still take my vitamins, supplements, and medications? Yes, definitely continue taking your medications. If you normally take them with food, just take them with your juice at your normal time. One word of caution: Grapefruit juice can interfere with the absorption of some medications. So check with your health care professional before taking any medication with any juice containing grapefruit. Also,

if you are taking blood thinners, anticoagulants, or have any kind of blood clotting issues, check with your doctor. The green juices have high levels of vitamin K, which is a natural clotting agent and can interfere with the action of anticlotting medications. In fact, as we mentioned in Chapter 1, anyone with any kind of health problem should check with their doctor before embarking on a Cleanse.

Can I exercise during my Cleanse? Absolutely! In fact, exercising is another way of cleansing, particularly if you sweat a lot. Our suggestion is that you drink a juice just before you head to the gym or out for your run, then another upon your return to replenish the energy you used during your workout. We also recommend that you put any super workouts on hold during your Cleanse. This is *not* the time to train for a marathon or take a boot camp class.

Can I have seltzer or sparkling water? We don't recommend it because they will make you gassy. But if they are the only nonjuice beverages you can drink, then they're better than nothing.

Can I drink Diet Coke? That's a solid "no." In addition to the gas issue, the sweetness will only make you crave sweet foods more than ever. It also contains caffeine and is a highly acidic food, upsetting the pH balance of your blood.

I have to travel. What should I do with my juice? You can't bring homemade juices with you since, as we noted earlier, their freshness is guaranteed for just a few minutes after you make them. So if you want to Cleanse while you're traveling, order your juices from us. You can put them into three-ounce containers and bring them on the plane or, if your flight is short, put them in a cooler with ice packs and check them with your luggage. We actually recommend cleansing during trips to counteract the toxins from airplanes and the stress from travel overall. Plus, if you're drinking water throughout your Cleanse, it can counteract the dehydration that often results from dry airplane air.

Can I sweeten my tea? If you must sweeten your tea, do it with a teaspoon or less of agave nectar, which is what we use in our packaged juices. Agave nectar is a natural sugar that is less likely to lead to a blood sugar spike.

My teeth need to gnaw on something…either gum or my colleague's arm. Can I chew gum during the Cleanse? Chewing gum contributes to gas in your system as well as "confusing" the digestive process. It makes your stomach think that food is coming when it isn't, so you have all these digestive enzymes released. If you must have something to chew, grab a few sticks of celery or the other foods we recommend on page 103.

I have a work meeting and I can't drink a juice during it. If I eat a light salad, will it totally mess up my Cleanse? This is not the end of the world and you'll be just fine. Try to stick to the foods listed on our cheat sheet on page 103 before you go all out. Our best recommendation is to schedule your Cleanse when your life is the least complicated.

I can't get the green juices down; I've tried everything…is it okay if I just skip them? Is it enough calories? Skip the green juice? No way. It's delicious and the workhorse of the Cleanse. Power through it; it's got all the good stuff. Good stuff means vitamins, minerals,

> nutrients, antioxidants, flavonoids, enzymes, and more. You could try adding some fresh-squeezed lemon juice or pouring the juice over ice. That often helps.

Now, we're not going to lie to you. The first day can be difficult. Or as one of our clients bluntly put it: "Honestly, the first day is *hell*! I feel constantly hungry and there is an inner war with one part of me asking, 'Why in the world are you doing this? Stop NOW!'"

Listen, if you feel so bad that you want to quit, then quit! Don't feel guilty—by no means should you feel like you failed. The fact that you got this far—the preparation phase and through the first day of the Cleanse—is something to be proud of. Just make sure you ease back into real food by following the advice in Chapter 6. Even one day without food has put your digestive system into slow mode; you don't want to rev it up too quickly or you may find yourself feeling nauseous and sick. And remember, you can always try a longer Cleanse another time! But guess what? Even if you decide to quit, you should try to at least incorporate a fresh juice or two into your day along with the rest of the solid food you eat. Keep those enzymes coming and it will be easier to digest your regular food.

But if you can stick with the Cleanse for even one more day, we guarantee the results will be worth it! And remember: Everyone's experience is different.

Here's what our client Syama had to say about her first Cleanse: "I am a very active person. I go out to dinners and parties almost every night, there is never enough time to get it all in. Having said that, I knew that there would be no perfect time to start a Cleanse and was a little worried about disrupting my lifestyle to do this. I decided to do it anyway and I was thoroughly impressed.

"I was never hungry. I went to the gym, met up with friends, and even sat in on a couple of lunches/dinners. I am a generally healthy person, but I definitely feel my skin looks great and I have now been off coffee for five days (a huge accomplishment). I'm now thinking of doing a 1-Day Cleanse once a month."

Some of our clients are like Syama, and say the juices alleviate their hunger just fine. Others are like Monica and find that around the second day the hunger hits. "I really had to pull everything out of me not to eat...once I had my fifth juice, I was good to go. The third day was a normal day. I could have definitely done five days."

And here's what another client wrote on her blog: "Yes, I was hungry. Yes, I cheated. And yes, I felt fine—better than fine even. I was most definitely hungry throughout all three days—I wasn't starving to the point I wanted to chew my own arm off, but I definitely wanted more. And on day two, I indulged in an apple and some almonds. Day three, I graduated to an apple, almonds, and some tortilla chips. Day three may have been my own fault. I took my favorite Sunday morning gym class, a mix of body sculpting and cardio. The class was probably too intense for someone who hadn't eaten (much) solid food in over forty-eight hours, hence the tortilla chips."

This woman didn't "cheat." She did what she had to in order to continue on the Cleanse. The overall benefits she received from managing to get through the three days far exceeded any "negatives" from a few tortilla chips and nuts! Remember our mantra...to each his or her own. Flexibility is key. Do what feels right for *you*.

If you are hungry, there are a few foods you can munch on (see "Cleanse Clients Ask..." on the next page). We also recommend tea. Lots and lots of tea. Herbs that help stem hunger include thyme, fennel, and mint. Wheatgrass is another option. Try brewing each or all into teas that you sip throughout the day, hot or cold. If you'd rather buy your teas ready-made, we recommend Adagio Teas, Harney & Sons, Yogi Tea, and Traditional Medicinals. All have websites from which you can order their products.

Cleanse Clients Ask...
I'm at the end of my first day of the Cleanse, and I just don't think I can continue. I'm dying for something to chew!

No worries! If you feel that you simply *must* chew, grab one of the following:

- A few celery stalks
- Half a sliced cucumber
- One-quarter mashed avocado with 1 tablespoon of lemon juice mixed in

One juice cleanser notes that sometimes just the simple of act of chewing makes a difference in how you feel and helps banish hunger pangs. "I think it's the act of chewing that makes the difference," she says. "I'm not sure that I'm really hungry because I drink as much juice as I want and it does fill up my stomach. Several times I've decided to fast, started on the juice and then eaten salads or fruit later in the day, and then gradually tapered off on the solid stuff."

Just remember that the less you consume, the faster you detox. The more solids that you introduce, the more you slow the detox process. We like to think of detoxing as a train—the fewer the passengers, the lighter the train and thus the faster it goes. Once you start putting people on the train, it slows down.

The same occurs with your body. When you are constantly ingesting, your body can't find the time or energy to detox. It's too busy and bogged down deal-ing with the incoming to focus on the outgoing.

However, if you're doing the Cleanse and are

experiencing numerous symptoms such as headaches, skin eruptions, nausea, etc., it could mean that your body has all the energy and time in the world to stir up that old stuff that has not been unearthed since you were eighteen. Once those toxins get stirred up, your body dumps everything into your bloodstream, where it is filtered by your detoxing organs and, hopefully, exits your body via sweat and urine.

So if you're experiencing these symptoms because you're detoxing too fast, try munching on a piece of cucumber or some celery to slow the train and, consequently, banish the uncomfortable symptoms.

Even putting some vegetables or fruits with the skin on into a blender—not a juicer—can help because the extra fiber and bulk "distract" your system from detoxing and focus it back on digesting, slowing the detox and moderating your symptoms.

Our main advice is to avoid acidic condiments such as vinegar or Tabasco, and stay away from any salt unless it's Celtic Sea Salt. These will interfere with your detox and digestion and make you feel, well, not good. You can, however, use apple cider vinegar, which actually has an alkaline effect on your blood.

DAY 2

At the end of day two I felt really energized so I took a yoga class then relaxed in the steam room after. After the steam, I exfoliated my face with a scrub. Maybe I was delirious from the lack of solid food, but I swear my acne was clearing up.

—SHERRIL

Finished my fifth juice. I still have a slight, dull headache, probably coffee deprivation. I'm not hungry and I'm really looking forward to my sixth juice with the cashew nut milk.

—MARQUINA

By Day 2, you should be well into the swing of the Cleanse. You'll feel lighter and, maybe, a little light-headed. You'll also find that if you're drinking enough fluid, you go to the bathroom nearly every hour. This is normal! Remember, don't worry if your urine is red; if you're drinking any juices made with beets, this is a common phenomenon.

You may also find that you actually feel *worse* today than you did yesterday. As one of our clients wrote on her blog about the second day of her Cleanse: "As the day wore on I was hungry and irritable. The cravings for food were so bad by the evening that if I'd been at a party or a dinner it might have been too much to take. For sure, I wouldn't have been pleasant to be around."

We tell you this to show you that feeling this way on Day 2 is perfectly normal. Don't think there's something wrong with you. If you feel like you can't take it anymore, but you really, really want to continue, try distracting yourself. Here are ten things to do instead of eating:

1. Take a walk.
2. Take a bubble bath (hard to eat in the bath).
3. Take a nap.
4. Take a shower and scrub your body—hard!
5. Have sex.
6. Get a mani-pedi (the smell in the nail salon will snap your appetite like a pretzel).
7. Go to the gym.
8. Go swimming.

9. Go to the florist shop and buy yourself some fabulous flow-
   ers (use the money you're saving by not eating out for three
   days!).
10. Go shopping.

Listen, the fact that you made it this far on the Cleanse is fantastic. As one of our clients noted: "After that first day it gets
easier. Much easier. Usually, sometime during the afternoon of
the second day I start to feel incredible: euphoric, light, almost
floating but in a good way. There's a real 'high' on the other side
of the suffering at the beginning. During this time I always regret
that we humans have to eat at all. It seems so much easier to just
skip the whole eating process—and it would certainly be more
pleasurable and save a lot of money and effort."

This is a good day to take your detox a step further. You can
do as Sherril did and spend some time in a steam room and exfo-
liate your face and body. Other suggestions:

- **Get a massage.** As we noted in Chapter 1, massage helps
  moves toxins out of your muscles into your bloodstream,
  where they can be excreted through urine.
- **Give yourself a full facial.** We're partial to masks that you
  leave on your face for fifteen minutes or so. They help draw
  out impurities and leave your skin glowing. (Of course, a spa
  facial is also an option!)
- **Try a colonic.** We talked about this in Chapter 1. You've
  probably heard enough to make up your mind already.
- **Detox your environment.** Now is a good time to clear out
  the clutter that makes your life toxic. Start with one closet or
  one drawer. You will be amazed at how liberating it is!

Keep in mind, however, that adding options such as massage and
sauna can intensify the detox symptoms because they stir up
more toxins. That's okay...just keep drinking your water and

taking care of yourself. And if you simply don't feel well, go to bed and rest. Even though you're giving your digestive system a rest, your body is still working hard to rid itself of the toxins emerging during the Cleanse.

I have reached euphoria. I'm not hungry. I have a spring in my step. I swear I can see more clearly. Like laser focus. Crazy. I'm not irritable. I called my cell phone company without becoming upset with the customer service rep. Wow.

—CATHY

Cleanse Clients Ask...
I've been on the fast for about thirty-six hours now and still haven't had a bowel movement. Is this normal?

Perfectly normal, particularly since there is far less fiber in the juices than in your regular diet and fiber is important in normal bowel movements. If you are uncomfortable, feel free to add one teaspoon of flaxseed oil to your juice or even take an herbal laxative such as Oxy-Oxc, Swiss Kriss, or Intestinal Formula #1.

Another option is a colonic (discussed in Chapter 1), or if you're comfortable doing it, self-administer an enema. Both are safe, gentle, and highly effective and we recommend them before, during, and after a Cleanse. The reason we keep pushing colonics is because it is so important that you keep eliminating while you cleanse. What are you eliminating? Toxins! If you don't get them out of your body, they can lead to some unwanted effects, such as bad breath, acne, and a weird rash.

Herbs such as dandelion root, rhubarb root,

cascara bark, and bayberry bark, taken as a supplement or brewed into a tea, can also help with constipation.

We also recommend probiotics for a healthy digestive system. They are the "good" bacteria, such as those found in unpasteurized yogurt or fermented vegetables, which help keep "bad" bacteria in check, reducing the risk of intestinal problems such as gas, bloating, constipation, and diarrhea. Take them in supplement form during the Cleanse; afterward, you can get them through unpasteurized yogurt.

HOW ARE YOU FEELING?

You may be surprised at what your body throws at you during a Cleanse. We heard of one woman who did an 11-Day Cleanse, and an itching on her cheek turned out to be a suture from a small surgery thirty years previous that made its way to the surface!

You may not have to worry about long-lost sutures, but you may be worrying about detox symptoms. Maybe you heard from friends who did hard-core fasts, or very minimalist juice cleanses, about terrible headaches, nausea, and shakiness, not to mention diarrhea or, on the other end, constipation.

It's doubtful you'll experience any of that on the Cleanse because it is not as extreme as other cleanses and fasts, so you're not detoxing as quickly, and because we provide such a nutrient-rich experience. However, simply eliminating most protein and fat can lead to some unique changes in your body as it works to cleanse itself. Here's what's normal....and what's not.

Keep in mind that everyone's symptoms will be different based on how long you cleanse for and how deep your toxic burden. The longer you detox, the more likely you are to experience these symptoms as long-buried toxins are dug up; shorter Cleanses tend to be less intense and you are less likely to experience most of the negative symptoms.

SYMPTOM	NORMAL	NOT NORMAL	COMMENTS
Headache	✓		Often results from caffeine withdrawal. Try a cup of green tea.
Mild acne or skin changes	✓		This is typical on the first or second day of the Cleanse as toxins leave your body through your skin.
Fatigue	✓		You may notice peaks and valleys of fatigue and energy. Nothing's wrong with a nap!
Unusual energy	✓		See above. Take advantage of these energy surges to start a new project or even simply clean out a closet (detox your closet, as it were).
Crankiness	✓		This is more typical the first day of the Cleanse when your blood sugar may be low, making you cranky.
Frequent urination	✓		This is a good thing! Go when you need to go and don't stop drinking water!
Strong body odor	✓		An unfortunate side effect of the detox. This is where a stint in the steam room can help.

SYMPTOM	NORMAL	NOT NORMAL	COMMENTS
Fainting		✓	Eat something light, such as a piece of fruit or a few crackers. See your health care professional.
Increased desire for and enjoyment of sex	✓		The extra energy and clarity you feel wakes up every part of your body. Every. Part.
Insomnia		✓	Actually, you should be sleeping better than ever. Instead of lying in bed awake with your mind racing, get up, brew a cup of camomile tea, and make of list of everything that's worrying you. Leave it on the table and go back to bed.
Increased productivity	✓		Extra energy, more focused thinking—you'll be amazed at how much you get done during the Cleanse.
Craving for alcohol, particularly wine	✓		This only occurs if you're a wine drinker to begin with. You'll have fewer cravings as your body becomes used to the fact that your nightly glass (glasses) of Chardonnay is missing in action.
Muscle cramps		✓	Could be low potassium. Eat a banana. And make sure you're getting enough fluid.

SYMPTOM	NORMAL	NOT NORMAL	COMMENTS
Glowing skin	✓		For the first time in years your skin will look the way nature intended...with no toxins to clog it up.
Irregular heartbeat		✓	Make sure you're drinking enough water and call your health care professional if it continues.
Red urine/ feces	✓	✓	If you did not drink a juice containing beets, see a health care professional.
Panic attack		✓	Breathe through it and call a health care professional.
Gas and bloating	✓		If you have gas or bloating, chew on aniseed, parsley, dill, ginger, or fennel, or steep the dried or fresh herbs in a cup of hot water for an "antigas" tea.
Constipation	✓		This is entirely normal, the result of a change in your diet. Keep drinking water and make sure you get a walk or other exercise into your day. Herbs that will help with constipation and stimulate your digestive system include cinnamon, spearmint, peppermint, ginger, burdock, licorice, cloves, and nutmeg.
Diarrhea/frequent bowel movements		✓	You're more likely to find you have fewer bowel movements, not more.

SYMPTOM	NORMAL	NOT NORMAL	COMMENTS
Weight loss	✓		You can expect to lose a few pounds of weight on the Cleanse, as discussed in Chapter 2.
Constantly thinking of food	✓		See our recommendations for distraction on page 103.

In addition to the physical changes listed in this table, we've also heard from clients about some other, uh, unique (at least to them) issues, actions, and thoughts that arise. Among them:

- Smiling at strangers
- Wishing for a longer Cleanse
- Crystal-clear eyes
- Holier-than-thou attitude
- Suddenly deciding to reprioritize your life
- Rethinking your eating habits
- Giving yourself an enema
- Getting a colonic
- Telling everyone about your colonic experience
- Going shopping for a new wardrobe to match the new you
- Adding up how much money you saved during the Cleanse because you didn't eat out, drink, etc.
- Looking at yourself naked in the mirror for long periods of time

I'm right smack in the middle of Day 2 of a 3-Day Cleanse. And really? Not so bad. I did cheat last night with some avocado and lemon juice (which tasted like the best thing ever), but half of that was because I just wanted to chew on something that didn't remind me of the green juice. As much as I hate the green juice, I can down it quickly and then be pleased with myself for taking in that much vegetation twice a day. And the cashew nut milk? Wow! That stuff is fantastic! (This is from someone who's usually a would-you-like-some-pie-with-your-whipped-cream kind of girl, know what I'm sayin'?)

—ALEXIS

DAY 3

Each Cleanse is different. Sometimes I feel very tired and sleep when my body tells me to. That's a sign that I was fatigued without even knowing it. Other times I have so much energy, I can't stay still! But most of all—and this is what I treasure—I feel euphoric! Light! Free!!! I get my best insights and ideas and creative inspiration. I love it!!

—PEGGY

Congratulations! You've made it to Day 3. As we said earlier, the majority of our clients do 3-Day Cleanses. But a good number of them also find that they don't want to stop! They want to continue on, many for two or more days. If you're feeling this way, go for it! All it takes is a quick trip to the grocery store or farmer's market for more produce.

But most people find that three days are just enough. They're ready for solid food, for a variety of flavors and textures…all the things that make eating so much fun. We're all for that. But just as we cautioned you not to jump into the Cleanse, we now caution you not to jump out. In the next chapter we show you how to slowly emerge from the Cleanse so you wake up your digestive system gently and avoid any negative effects.

For now, how about a few words from Alexis, one of our Cleanse clients, about how her Cleanse changed her. By the end of the second day, she wrote us, she had:

- Cleaned out her fridge "big time. There are lots of foods that will never return to my home."
- Consumed more vegetables in the past thirty-six hours than she'd eaten in the past year.
- Rediscovered "the awesomeness that is avocado."
- Seriously began rethinking her overall diet.

She was also happy to report that she did *not*:

- Daydream about cheeseburgers.
- Freak out and gorge herself on queso.
- Break out, nor did she have any GI "episodes."
- Have an epiphany and decide to become a vegan.

Her conclusion? "Overall, this has been a most doable experience. I will definitely recommend it to friends, and will almost certainly be back the next time I feel like renovating/redecorating."

SHORTER? LONGER?

We talked quite a bit about the benefits of even a 1-Day Cleanse and the amazing benefits of a long-term Cleanse (five or more days). Just remember that your experience and benefits fall along a continuum. The shorter the Cleanse, the less likely you are to experience negative physical effects; the longer the Cleanse, the more likely you are. However, the shorter the Cleanse, the less deep detoxing you're doing; the longer the Cleanse, the more deeply the cleaning occurs.

Bottom line, however: Do what's right for you!

CHAPTER 6

After the Cleanse

My first Cleanse was terrific and I experienced everything that you indicated I would. I felt great, had such an increased energy level, lost five pounds, and even my skin glowed. Then I didn't follow the steps to come out of the Cleanse. I attended two gala events in a row, just two days after the Cleanse. Besides the Chardonnay, I ate appetizers, fish, veggies, and all sorts of other things that, just as you warned me, did not sit well with me. Oh my goodness, I was miserable for a number of days (as you can imagine).

—Sarah

So...how did your Cleanse go? More important, how do you *feel*? Whether you stayed on it for one day or five days, made it through with *just* juice or added some of the solid foods allowed, we're sure you feel...well, *cleaner.* Lighter. Fresher. Maybe you discovered some truths about yourself you weren't aware of. Like the fact that you actually *like* green juice! Maybe the focus on how you were feeling physically made you realize that you actually hadn't been feeling very good lately. And that maybe the junk you've been putting into your body isn't really the way to go.

Here's what one of our clients wrote: "As a 32-year-old mother of two, I have suffered from chronic sinusitis and a deficient immune system for quite some time—no energy, a regular at the doctor's office...an all-around slug. Additionally, before starting the Cleanse, it took me a pot of coffee each morning to even open my eyelids wide enough to drive carpool. NO MORE!! I am happy to say that I lost enough weight to warrant throwing a 'Welcome Home' party for my waistline, I now no longer need caffeine, I have the mental clarity of a Mensa member (well, almost!), and I'm rolling with the energy of a 16-year-old! I feel like Superwoman and I may just order myself a cape."

We received this from Doug (for those of you who are wondering: Yes! Men do the Cleanse, too!): "I'm stunned at the amount of energy I have, the clarity with which I'm able to think, and, mostly, the realization of how much garbage I was putting into my system. There are several people in my office who have commented that I actually look healthier. Thanks so much. I truly feel like this is one of those moments in my life that I will never forget because of the impact it has and will continue to have on my health."

A common story is the one here from Suz, who, after completing her Cleanse, wrote on her blog: "I am not craving dairy/sugar like I was five days ago. Which is good because I really shouldn't eat those due to food allergies/intolerances. So overall, I feel better and less bloated. I also feel more in control of eating. Just today I realized I tend to have a 'habit' of snacking during activities (blogging, reading, watching TV) when I'm not actually hungry. So before I fall back into those habits I'm going to make an effort to stick to planned meals and snacks and not eat a bag of popcorn just because we popped in this week's Netflix."

We'll get into the post-Cleanse life in the next chapter. For now, we want to talk reentry—the five days after your Cleanse when you reintroduce solid food. This is still a time of cleansing, with the reintroduction of solid food forming a base to remove additional toxins from your body via your digestive system. So don't treat this time too lightly.

Instead, we recommend you do what Kathy did after her Cleanse: "Today is the first day after the Cleanse and I am at work eating my fresh fruit with some lettuce and cucumber planned for later along with a lot of water," she wrote us. "Once again, I feel amazing. I feel as though I have taken a wonderful bath from the inside out, if that makes sense."

As with the pre-Cleanse, you should *not,* repeat *not,* dive right in with a cheeseburger and fries. Just reread the quote from Sarah that opens this chapter.

Remember: Your digestive system has been on hiatus for several days. Just as it's not healthy for you to floor the gas and make your car go from 0 to 60 in 10 seconds, neither is it healthy for you to "floor" your digestive system with a heavy meal of difficult-to-process foods. It also won't feel good. And really, do you want a wave of nausea overcoming you on your first post-Cleanse day? Along with nausea, abruptly awakening your digestive system could also lead to stomach cramps and bloating.

Instead, we recommend you *eeeeaaassse* into eating with the following schedule:

Day 1 post-Cleanse: A few pieces of fruit spread throughout the day or some fresh-squeezed nonpasteurized juice (green, citrus, or fruit). Just be sure to dilute the juice with water.

Day 2 post-Cleanse: Raw or lightly steamed vegetables, e.g., spinach and broccoli. Avoid the starchier vegetables such as carrots, beets, squash, and potatoes. You may also have a raw green leafy salad with some vegetables.

Day 3 post-Cleanse: Green salads should be your staple at this point. If you're craving more sustenance, you may choose a small portion of plain brown rice or a yam or sweet potato.

Day 4 post-Cleanse: If you eat poultry, you may incorporate some now or some lightly steamed or poached fish, with veggies and a salad, of course!

Day 5 post-Cleanse: Denser foods such as red meat and processed foods can now reenter your diet—if you want!

The most impressive thing about the 3-Day Cleanse is this:
You honestly do not feel like you are fasting for three days.
And overall, I'm thrilled with the results. I'm definitely thinner,
especially in my waist. In fact, I'm not sure it's ever been this
chiseled. On the less vain front, I feel less rundown and a nagging
cold/allergies I've had most of the year are completely gone.

—MARIE

MOVING FROM CLEANSING TO FOOD COMBINING

Now, wouldn't you like to retain that great feeling and healthier digestive system for more than just a few days? Then we recommend you follow the philosophy of food combining. We explain it in more detail in Chapter 7, but we wanted to introduce the basic rules in this chapter, since your post-Cleanse reentry program is based on these principles.

Food combining is a system designed to improve digestion over the long term—not just after a Cleanse. The theory behind food combining, which dates back to the nineteenth century, is that specific foods require specific enzymes for the most efficient and complete digestion. For instance, lipases break down fats only. Not proteins, not carbohydrates. The quicker the enzymes can break down the food into its nutritional components, the less time it spends in your stomach and the less likely you are to experience gas, bloating, and constipation.

We will get more into the details in the next chapter when we talk about the long-term post-Cleanse life, but here are the basics:

1. Eat proteins and carbohydrates separately.
2. Eat only one "concentrated" protein at each meal. A concentrated protein is a food that is primarily protein, such as eggs, meat, poultry, and fish.
3. Treat juices, whether vegetable or fruit, as whole foods, not drinks.
4. Have dessert. Just make sure it's not fruit. Dark chocolate is the best.
5. Eat your food warm or at room temperature. Cold food inhibits digestion.
6. Eat fruit alone on an empty stomach as a "fruit meal." And don't eat it in between meals unless your stomach is empty.

7. Do not eat sweet and acid fruits together (more on the difference in the next chapter).

Now turn to Chapter 7 to learn how to live the rest of your post-Cleanse life and how to make the Cleanse a regular part of your life rather than just a one-time-only experience.

3-Day Cleanse Tip

It's easier to follow your post-Cleanse diet if you refrain from dining out or having dinner with friends for at least the first couple of days. Explain to them that it's important that you reintegrate food into your life by ounces, not pounds, and that you'll be far better company for a meal in just a few days.

The Post-Cleanse Meal Plan

DAY 1 POST-CLEANSE

Breakfast
Fresh fruit—papaya or pineapple

Lunch
Grapefruit Avocado Salad (recipe page 153)

Snack
Fresh fruit

Dinner
Roasted Red Pepper Soup (recipe page 143)

DAY 2 POST-CLEANSE

Breakfast

Smoothie of your choice from the recipes beginning on page 207

Lunch

Mango Lettuce Wrap (recipe page 176)

Snack

Sesame Dip with cut veggies (recipe page 196)

Dinner

Spaghetti Squash (recipe page 178) topped with store-bought organic pasta sauce

DAY 3 POST-CLEANSE

Breakfast

Sprouted grain toast with almond butter

Lunch

Fresh Fava and Escarole Salad with shaved Parmesan (recipe page 159)

Snack

Sweet Potato and Beetroot Crisps (recipe page 197)

Dinner

Oven-Roasted Tilapia (recipe page 182)

Marinated Kale with Tahini Dressing (recipe page 173)

CHAPTER 7

Cleansing for the Long Term

Truth be told, the hardest part is coming off the Cleanse. In some ways, it's much easier not to eat at all! But once those taste buds reawaken, the simplest food tastes marvelous. I could actually taste the sugar in broccoli!

—Carol

As we discussed in the previous chapter, it *is* possible to continue the wonderful feeling you have after a Cleanse nearly indefinitely. It has to do with changing the way that you eat.

We both follow the food combining principles described in the previous chapter, although Zoë has been doing it far longer than Erica. She used to eat everything, including lots of meat. Her philosophy: "The more I could combine and mix together, the better." But she used to feel horrible after every meal. How horrible she didn't realize until she changed how she ate and finally felt good.

She became a raw foodist, but that didn't help. She now knows that's because she knew nothing about food combining or how long certain foods took to digest. She didn't know that different foods call for different digestive enzymes, that they are meant to work independently, and that when they're forced to meet, it's an all-out war.

For instance, she learned that starches are digested by the enzyme amylase; that protein requires protease; that fats require lipase; and that various carbohydrates require specific enzymes to break them down into glucose, depending on what type of sugar they are.

Then she learned that every food has its own specific transit time and that certain foods take longer to digest than others. Liquid is quickest and animal protein takes the longest.

That made her realize that if she ate fruit for dessert, it would zip right through her system but would eventually get blocked by whatever protein she ate as the main course. What happens next is, well... gross. The fruit sits there on top of the protein and ferments, creating gas in your system.

Thus, we now know that one of the greatest myths in nutrition is that eating fruit for dessert is healthy. Even some of the strictest raw foodists believe this, those who don't know the "rule of transit."

Today, we always think about how long it will take a food to go through our system before exiting, and what potential "roadblocks" might occur along the way.

Once you know what category your food falls into, food combining becomes very simple to follow...

Nonstarchy vegetables: asparagus, beet greens, broccoli, Brussels sprouts, cabbage, celery, chard, chicory, collards, cucumber, dandelion, eggplant, endive, escarole, garlic, green beans, kale, kohlrabi, leeks, lettuce, onions, parsley, radishes, scallions, spinach, sprouts, squash, sweet pepper, Swiss chard, tomatoes, turnips, watercress, zucchini

Mildly starchy vegetables: artichokes, beets, carrots, cauliflower, corn, peas

Acid fruit: blackberry, grapefruit, lemon, lime, orange, pineapple, plum, pomegranate, raspberry, sour apple, strawberry

Subacid fruit: apple, apricot, blueberry, cherry, kiwi, mango, papaya, peach, pear, plum

Sweet fruit: bananas, dried fruits, dates, grapes, papaya, persimmon

Melon: cantaloupe, casaba, Crenshaw, honeydew, papaya melon, Persian melon, musk melon, watermelon

Proteins: cheese, coconut, eggs, fish, meat, milk, nuts, olives, poultry, seeds, soybeans, yogurt

Fats and oils: avocado, butter, corn oil, cream, lard, nut oils, olive oil, safflower oil, soy oil, sesame oil

Carbohydrates: beans, bread, cereals, grains, lentils, potatoes, pumpkin, split peas, squash (acorn, banana, Hubbard)

The Food Combining Cheat Sheet

If the food combining rules on page 120 are too complicated, just remember this simple formula:

protein + carbohydrate or fat = poor

That means forget about beans and rice, steak and potatoes, tuna noodle casserole, and skip the lemon butter on your fish.

carbohydrate + fat = good

nonstarchy vegetables + fat *or* carbohydrate *or* protein = excellent!

mildly starchy vegetables + protein *or* carbohydrate = good

Do not combine fruits from different categories, and always eat fruits *alone*: no sugar on your grapefruit!

THE ACID-BASE DIET AND OTHER STEPS FOR GOOD DIGESTION

Food combining has its roots in the whole idea of maintaining a proper pH (acid-base) balance in your gut and in your blood. The modern American diet generates a significant amount of acid, requiring that your bones release calcium to make your blood more alkaline and to bring the acid-base levels back into balance. This, of course, can weaken bone.

Common sources of acid in our diet include red meat, fish, chicken, eggs, cheese, peanuts and most nuts, beans, peas and other legumes, and grains. See what we mean when we suggest you limit your protein intake? All you need is more than 75 grams (about 3 ounces) of protein a day to upset the acid-base balance. Although the average American gets about 70 grams...many of us get more. In fact, the highest rate of hip fractures in women occurs in countries in which women eat the highest amounts of animal protein!

To counter acid, you need potassium and magnesium, ideally from plant-based foods. Our juices and other recipes in this book are all designed to maintain an acid-base balance; the rest of your diet should, too.

Other tips for proper digestion...

Chew starches slowly. The salivary enzyme amylase is critical for proper starch digestion. The longer the starchy food is in contact with your saliva, the less work your gastric enzymes have to do. That's why rapidly swallowing poorly chewed food can make you feel sick.

Stick with whole grains and other high-fiber foods. Fiber not only helps prevent constipation, but also slows the absorption of sugar and fat, preventing the post-meal spike in insulin that can leave you feeling light-headed and cranky after a high-carbohydrate-only meal.

Avoid processed foods whenever possible. They are often a conglomeration of protein, carbohydrates, fats, etc., and also contain a variety of different sugars, each of which requires different enzymes to digest. For instance, sucrase breaks down sucrose (made from sugar beets or sugar cane) into glucose and fructose; maltase breaks down maltose (found in grains) into glucose; isomaltase breaks down maltose and isomaltose; and lactase breaks down lactose (found in dairy).

Plus, many processed foods are simply *loaded* with sugar. Take a look at the ingredient list for Kellogg's® Pop-Tarts® Frosted

S'mores and you'll see six different kinds of sugar: sugar, high-fructose corn syrup, dextrose, corn syrup, corn syrup solids, lactose (a sugar found in milk), and brown sugar. Also watch out for the word "sorbitol" on the label. This is an alcohol sugar often added to "diabetic" or "unsweetened" products. It's still a sugar; it just takes longer to be absorbed into your bloodstream.

If you've been in the habit of dining on these types of foods, the post-Cleanse time might be the best time to cut yourself loose. Someone we know who does juice cleanses as well as fasts told us, "It's easy to not eat junk after a fast—or at least, it's easy for me. I feel so great that I don't want to disturb this feeling, and the thought of something heavy like cheese or a burger or even a dessert is simply repugnant. It's not at all like, 'Whew, that's over. Let's chow down.' A piece of fruit seems like an effort and almost overwhelming. In fact, for several days after a juice fast I eat very little—out of choice, not discipline. Naturally, the eating routine overtakes me again and I get back to normal. I'm regretful, though. The 'high' is so incredible that I'd really like to live that way."

High-Fructose Corn Syrup

A word about high-fructose corn syrup (HFCS). We talked a bit about this in Chapter 1, but it's worth repeating. This manufactured sweetener has become ubiquitous in processed foods, even in things you wouldn't think need extra sweetening such as pasta sauce, breads, and salsa. Studies find that adults can handle only a limited amount of fructose, particularly the type produced with corn syrup. Just 24 ounces of soda (which contains about 50 grams of fructose, usually in the form of HFCS), is enough to produce abdominal pain, bloating, gas, and constipation.

Cut back on protein. Most Americans get far more protein in their diets than they need. We need only about a third of a gram of protein for every pound of body weight. So if you weigh 150 pounds, you need about 54 grams of protein. Yet the *average* American gets about 70 grams of protein a day; since that's an average, many of us get far more. As noted earlier, high-protein diets tip the acid-base balance of your blood out of balance into a highly acidic state, forcing your bones to release calcium in order to reduce the acidity and weakening your bones. High-protein diets also put stress on your kidneys, increase the risk of high blood pressure, and, studies show, can increase your risk of certain cancers.

When choosing your protein, choose vegetable over animal. For instance, you might get 38 grams of protein in a 6-ounce piece of steak, but you'll also get 44 grams of fat, much of them artery-clogging saturated fat. Two cups of cooked lentils provide nearly the same amount of protein but with less than 1 gram of fat.

Choose the right cheese. We love cheese. Yes, it's difficult to digest, can cause serious intestinal gas and bloating, and is definitely not on the path of a low-fat food (unless you choose low-fat cheese). However, there are varying degrees in the land of dairy and, as we said before, you have to live your life.

We prefer raw cheeses. Unlike pasteurized cheeses, raw cheeses contain live enzymes that are beneficial for healthy digestion. We also try to stay away from cheese made from cow milk, which we find most difficult to digest, and choose those made from sheep or goat milk.

Get the right kind of flavoring. We recommend two in particular: Bragg Liquid Aminos and sea salt. Bragg Liquid Aminos is a savory yet low-sodium alternative to salt and soy sauce. Derived from soybeans, the flavoring contains sixteen amino acids with no preservatives, gluten, alcohol, chemicals, or artificial coloring. We consider it the best, most natural flavoring we can recommend to our clients.

We choose sea salt over regular table salt for numerous reasons. Sea salt has larger crystals, so you can get more flavor with less sodium. It also has no added iodine, which can give salt an "off" taste (a much better source of iodine is sea vegetables such as dried seaweed). In addition, sea salt doesn't contain any additives to prevent clumping. Sea salt is derived from evaporated seawater (duh!), while table salt is mined from mineral deposits. We just think sea salt tastes better! Our favorite is Celtic Sea Salt, which we also think has energizing priorities. We like to put it into a pepper grinder and grind it over our food. Again, you'll use less.

The "New You" Shopping List

As you embrace this new way of eating, you will find yourself reaching for different products in grocery stores. Here is what we consider the essential staples, or the "what I have in my kitchen at all times" list. All are available at health food stores and stores such as Whole Foods; even most "regular" supermarkets stock these items today.

Nama Shoyu (raw soy sauce)
Bragg Liquid Aminos
sprouted grains
74% dark chocolate
apple cider vinegar
Celtic Sea Salt
cold-pressed extra virgin olive oil

FROM THIS DAY FORWARD

Now let's talk a bit about where the Cleanse comes into the rest of your life. As we hope you've already learned, cleansing is no longer about zoning out in a drum circle while sipping lemon juice and cayenne pepper. It's not about taking off for a spa and then returning to your usual unhealthy diet and lifestyle once you get back home. It is not extreme. The 3-Day Cleanse is about detoxing regularly, when you need to, in a way that suits your own body—all while carrying on with life as you know it.

Another good rule of thumb for when to cleanse is whenever you experience fatigue, a general lack of energy, sleeplessness, anxiety, depression, or digestive problems, and at the first sign of a cold or other illness or infection. Also consider cleansing when you get a bad report from the doctor. As one of our clients wrote us: "My husband just came back from the doctor—his cholesterol has dropped 30 points in the last two months since he started doing the 3-Day Cleanse regularly!"

Although we don't recommend juice-only Cleanses if you have diabetes (unless your doctor gives you the green light), we do recommend them if you are having blood sugar issues, i.e., slightly higher-than-normal blood sugar caused by insulin resistance.

Seasonally, spring and autumn are the best times of the year to cleanse. But there are no bad times.

Bottom line: We strongly suggest a minimum of three days a month to give your body the proper rest and recovery time it needs to maintain optimum health. Make it a healthy habit—the immune system loves a consistent schedule.

We also recommend "mini-Cleanses." For instance:

- BluePrintCleanse's Juice 'Til Dinner™. Once a week, drink only BluePrintCleanse juices—your own or purchased—until dinner and then dine on a light salad or any of the recipes coded 1 or 2.

- Add one or more of the juices to your regular diet to supplement with healthy enzymes and antioxidants when you're *not* cleansing.

You can also take cleansing on the road. For instance, when you travel, you can either have juices delivered right to your hotel room or ship your own juices in ice packs along with luggage. Or at the very least, you can follow a raw food diet using the food combining methods we described earlier.

Other "real-life" scenarios:

Going out to dinner with friends. Maintaining your commitment to food combining is relatively easy in restaurants...these days nearly everything is à la carte anyway. And a simple salad and a piece of fish (steamed or broiled with no fat) make a healthy, light meal that won't throw your digestive system into overload. Or if you want the pasta, ask about whole wheat and swap out the protein for veggies. And what about the cheese plate at the end of the night? Let's just say some things are sacred.

Having dinner at a friend's house. Just choose the foods you know will work for you. But remember: Flexibility is key. Discarding the food combining principles in order to be a good guest is no big deal! Just pick them up the next day or, even better, make the following day a juice-only day!

A cocktail party. Limit your alcohol intake to one drink, or sip plain water with lime. You can munch on raw vegetables (but skip the dip) or, conversely, pieces of pure protein, such as steamed shrimp or raw oysters.

Sporting events. First, see if you can bring your own food in. A bunch of raw carrots to munch on or some cut-up fruit would be great. Conversely, some almonds or cashews can provide a good alternative to the more-difficult-to-digest peanuts.

As a last resort, think simple: Ask for a club soda from the fountain and munch on some plain popcorn.

Dessert and snacks. Everyone needs a little sweetness in their life. Get it with dark chocolate that is at least 74% cocoa.

This is chocolate in its purest form, which digests neutrally, so it can follow any meal. The goal is to skip out on the processed sugar, cream, and other things you can't pronounce that exist in milk chocolate.

We hope that by providing you with options—rather than hard-and-fast rules that tell you only what you *can't* do—you can find a way to incorporate a bit of our philosophy into your own. The final message we want to leave you with here is that you don't have to change your entire life or make major sacrifices to do something good for your body and to feel better than you did before. It's about understanding where you are, and what small improvements you can make from there.

Work hard. Play hard. Cleanse. Repeat.

Cheers!

THE RECIPES

These recipes are all either raw or partially raw, and we have coded them according to where they fit into your prep and transition process, both before and after a Cleanse. The key to remember is that the preparation into a Cleanse and the transition out should be a gradual process, so your body can slowly adjust to the minimal digestive effort that the Cleanse allows. If you go immediately from dense and poorly combined meals, even ones that seem "healthy," straight into the raw juices, your body will think it's still supposed to be in heavy digestion mode and likely put forth more effort than necessary in breaking down the juice, resulting in feelings of nausea and hunger. Example: Brown rice or whole wheat pasta, particularly with a protein such as tofu or soy, is far too dense for the night before a Cleanse. Enjoy things like this about three days out, but not immediately before or after (and skip the tofu/soy altogether to avoid the difficult starch + protein combination).

You'll notice that there aren't a ton of recipes for sweets or desserts. This is for two reasons: Um, you're *cleansing* and trying to get the sweet stuff *out* of your system! Besides, our favorite little sweet indulgence is much more easily purchased than made: dark chocolate! Anything with a 70% or higher cacao content digests quite simply and tastes amazing, to boot! The second reason is that the best desserts that fit into the raw guidelines take a *lot* of time and are very labor intensive—we're trying to make your life easier, not have you waiting over a bowl of sprouted groats until the moment you can make grawnola, etc. But power to the peeps who will make them for you. Support them at your local health food store! A last note on desserts—please resist the urge to follow a savory and satisfying meal with a piece of fruit. This is food combining 101: Fruit after a meal is a big no-no! Go for the chocolate—yes, you have the green light.

Each recipe will be coded with a 1, 2, or 3. These numbers correspond to the day in your prep/transition process that it is okay to have these ingredients. Since transitioning in and out of a cleanse should be a gradual process, the higher the number, the farther away from your Cleanse it should be incorporated.

Soups

Cucumber and Corn Soup | 1

This soup has a delicious and fresh flavor with a hint of Southwestern spice. Season it to your taste if you like a little more heat!

1 cup fresh corn kernels (from 1 ear of corn)
1/4 cup onion, chopped
1/2 cup seedless or English cucumber, diced
1 teaspoon fresh mint, chopped
1 teaspoon dill, chopped
1 tablespoon extra virgin olive oil
1/2 teaspoon sea salt
2 teaspoons lime juice
1 tablespoon water
pinch chili powder
1/4 ripe avocado, pitted, peeled, and cubed

Combine all the ingredients except the avocado in a bowl. Set aside about 1/4 of the combination. Blend 3/4 of the mixture until smooth, then pour into serving dishes. Add the avocado to the unblended mixture and gently mix in. Add the mixture to the serving dishes. Garnish with black pepper and serve.

Gazpacho | 1
MAKES 2-4 SERVINGS

No fussing with recipe translation here—gazpacho is the ulti-mate in raw! Fresh and filling with a touch of crunch, it's a great starter to any meal or a perfect summer meal on its own. Sherry vinegar can be substituted for white wine vinegar for a richer flavor.

1 English cucumber, peeled, seeded, and diced

1/2 orange pepper, seeded and diced

1/2 yellow pepper, seeded and diced

3 medium tomatoes, seeded and diced

1-2 tablespoons white wine vinegar (to taste)

1-2 cloves garlic

3 tablespoons extra virgin olive oil

2 teaspoons sea salt

1/2 avocado, peeled and diced (garnish)

black pepper to taste

Place 1/2 cup cucumber and 1/2 cup bell peppers in a medium-sized bowl. Place the remaining ingredients except the avocado in a food processor and pulse until smooth. Add to the diced ingredients and stir to combine. Garnish with the avocado, a drizzle of olive oil, and fresh-ground black pepper.

Roasted Red Pepper Soup | 1
MAKES 1-2 SERVINGS (16 OUNCES)

This beautiful and vibrant soup is loaded with antioxidants and lycopene (good for the prostate), and is equally delicious served warm or chilled. You can play with the flavor by finishing it with more chopped basil for an Italian-themed menu, or adding cilantro and a dash of cumin for a more Southwestern flavor.

1/4 cup raw cashews, soaked 1-2 hours
1/2 cup water
1/2 teaspoon sea salt
black pepper
3/4 teaspoon fresh lemon juice
1/2 teaspoon agave
1 pinch cayenne
1 pinch red chili flakes
1 cup roasted red bell peppers
1 tablespoon extra virgin olive oil
1 large basil leaf, chopped

Blend all the ingredients, except the basil, in a blender until smooth. Heat the mixture in a saucepan until slightly warmed. Pour into serving bowls, garnish with chopped basil, and serve.

For easy roasted bell peppers, halve and seed two red peppers, brush with olive oil, and place under a broiler for 5-7 minutes, until the skin is slightly blackened. Use a sharp knife to remove the skin.

Carrot Ginger Soup with Coriander | 2
MAKES 1-2 SERVINGS (16 OUNCES)

This is a quick and delicious soup that's great for a busy week-night dinner. Serve warm or chilled, depending on the season!

- 2 tablespoons extra virgin olive oil
- 1/2 cup yellow onion, chopped
- 1/4 cup fresh ginger, peeled and chopped
- 4 cups carrots, chopped
- 3 cups organic vegetable stock
- 1/4 teaspoon ground coriander
- sea salt and black pepper to taste

Add the olive oil, onion, and ginger to a saucepan over medium heat. Sauté 5 minutes until the onions are translucent. Add the carrots and vegetable stock; simmer and cover 30 minutes. Place in a blender and blend until smooth. Add salt and pepper to taste and blend until well combined.

Cauliflower Soup with Watercress | 2

This is a fantastic fall or winter soup meal—the pureed cauli-flower makes it hearty and filling and the watercress adds a nice note of clean flavor.

- 1 tablespoon extra virgin olive oil
- 1/4 yellow onion, chopped
- 1 tablespoon shallot, minced
- 1/2 head cauliflower, chopped (13 ounces)

1 bunch (6 ounces) fresh watercress, chopped and stems
   removed

2 cups organic vegetable broth (*not* made with tomato paste)

³/₄ teaspoon sea salt

black pepper to taste

1 tablespoon Nama Shoyu or Bragg Liquid Amino

1 teaspoon fresh lemon juice

Heat the olive oil in a heavy pot, and sauté the onions and shallot until translucent, about 5 minutes. Add the cauliflower and broth, bring to a boil, then turn heat to low, cover. Simmer 45 minutes. Add watercress and simmer 5 minutes, uncovered. Add remaining ingredients and stir. Place in a blender or use a hand blender and blend until smooth. Serve.

Chilled Cucumber Soup with Macadamia Cream | 2 (can be a 1 without the Macadamia Cream)
MAKES 1-2 SERVINGS (10 OUNCES)

This velvety soup is a great first course for an elegant dinner. Swirl in the Macadamia Cream (see recipe on page 167) with a spoon and sprinkle with fresh dill for a beautiful presentation. Make sure you plan ahead to give yourself at least an hour to soak the macadamias.

2 cups English (seedless) cucumbers, peeled and chopped
   (about 1 large)

2 tablespoons scallions, chopped

1 teaspoon lemon juice

1 teaspoon fresh dill, chopped

¹/₄ teaspoon sea salt

black pepper to taste

2 tablespoons extra virgin olive oil

2 tablespoons water

Blend all the ingredients until smooth. Pour into serving dishes and add a dollop of Macadamia Cream.

Cream of Broccoli Soup | 2
MAKES 16 OUNCES

Yep, you heard it. Cream of Broccoli. *You will be shocked at how delicious this tastes without using a drop of dairy.*

1 head broccoli, chopped into bite-size florets

1 ¹/₂ cups water

1 cup raw cashews, soaked 1 hour

¹/₈ teaspoon nutmeg

1 teaspoon sea salt

black pepper to taste

1 clove garlic

1 ¹/₂ teaspoons fresh lemon juice

¹/₈ teaspoon ground mustard seed

1 tablespoon extra virgin olive oil

¹/₂ teaspoon dried thyme

Bring 1 inch of water to a boil in a saucepan and add the broccoli; cover and reduce heat to medium; cook 6–7 minutes. Remove the broccoli as soon as it can be pierced by a fork. Drain the soaking water from the cashews; place the cashews in a high-speed blender with the nutmeg, sea salt, black pepper, garlic, lemon juice, mustard seed, and olive oil. Blend until smooth. Add the broccoli and pulse until the broccoli is chunky.

Add the mixture to a saucepan with the dried thyme. Turn the heat to medium and simmer for 5 minutes, stirring frequently. Serve.

Curried Butternut Squash Soup | 2
MAKES 4 CUPS

The curry in this soup balances out the sweetness of the squash and carrots for an exotic and rich flavor.

1 medium butternut squash, peeled, seeded, and chopped into
  1-inch cubes (about 6 cups)
1/2 teaspoon sea salt
4 tablespoons extra virgin olive oil
1 cup carrot juice (about 3 carrots)
2 tablespoons shallots, chopped (1 small shallot)
1 1/2 teaspoons sea salt
black pepper to taste
1 1/2 teaspoons red curry powder
2 tablespoons lime juice
2 teaspoons ginger, peeled and chopped
pinch cayenne
1 teaspoon chili powder

Preheat oven to 400°. Toss the butternut squash, salt, and olive oil together. Place in a baking dish and bake for 20–30 minutes until the squash can be pierced with a fork. Remove from heat and add to a blender with the remaining ingredients. Blend until smooth and serve warm.

Black Bean and Kale Soup | 3

MAKES 4 CUPS

You can probably tell by now that we're huge fans of kale, but it's a mystery green for many people when it comes to eating it rather than just juicing it. Its rich flavor and texture are ideal for a hearty soup like this one. Packed with vitamins K, A, and C and phytonutrients, which aid in the cleansing process by signaling our genes to increase production of enzymes involved in detoxification.

1 cup dried black beans—require soaking overnight so plan ahead!

1 tablespoon extra virgin olive oil

1/2 cup red onion, chopped (1 small red onion)

3 cloves garlic, minced

2 portabella mushrooms, stemmed and diced

2 teaspoons parsley, chopped

2 teaspoons jalapeño pepper, seeded and minced

1 teaspoon sea salt

4 1/2 cups warm water

2 cups kale, stems removed and roughly torn (8 stalks)

1 medium tomato, chopped

2 tablespoons Nama Shoyu

black pepper to taste

To cook beans:

Rinse the beans and place in a saucepan with 3 cups water. Bring to a boil and let boil for 2 minutes. Remove from heat and allow to sit, covered, for 24 hours.

For soup:

In a pot, heat the olive oil over medium heat; add the onion and garlic and cook until the onion is lightly browned, 8–10 minutes. Add the mushrooms, parsley, jalapeño, and a pinch of salt; cook, stirring often, until the mushrooms are tender, 5–6 minutes. Add 2 cups water; reduce to simmer, cover, and cook about 5 minutes. Add the kale, cover, and cook until wilted, about 2 minutes. Add the tomato, beans, and Nama Shoyu; cook (covered) for 20 minutes. Season with the remaining salt and pepper, and stir well to combine before serving.

Split Pea Soup | 3
MAKES 20 OUNCES

Thick and hearty, this is pure comfort food. A pot of this on the stove smells just like it did in Grandma's kitchen!

1/2 cup white or yellow onions, minced

1 clove garlic, minced

1 1/2 teaspoons extra virgin olive oil

1/2 teaspoon sea salt

black pepper to taste

1/2 cup carrots, diced (1 carrot)

3/4 cup dried split green peas

3 cups low-sodium vegetable stock (*not* made with tomato puree)

1 cup water

1 teaspoon parsley, chopped

1 1/2 tablespoons Bragg Liquid Aminos

Rinse the peas and drain; set aside. In a pot, heat the olive oil over medium heat. Add the onions, garlic, salt, and pepper;

sauté until the onions are translucent (approx. 3–5 minutes). Add the carrots, stock, and half of the split peas; simmer uncovered for 15 minutes. Add the remaining peas and water, cover, and continue to simmer for 45–50 minutes until the peas are soft. Add the parsley and Bragg's; stir in and season with more salt and pepper if desired. Remove from heat and serve.

Salads

This section includes a wide range of salads that go way beyond your basic mixed lettuces with tomatoes and cucumbers (not that there's anything wrong with that, we've got one of those, too!). Okay, so yes, we're total salad snobs, but for good reason! A well-composed salad is actually something to be appreciated. Too often a simple salad can become overcomplicated by too many ingredients or the wrong balance of flavors and textures, or could be vastly improved with a different dressing. For that reason, each salad is recommended with a particular dressing. Feel free to mix and match, but really, just trust us on this one.

Grapefruit Avocado Salad | 1
MAKES 2–4 SERVINGS

It's best to use a soft-leaf lettuce in this salad, as a crunchy one can overpower the balance. Try Bibb (aka Boston or butter lettuce) if red leaf is not available. This is great with any citrusy vinaigrette—we've paired it here with one using the mellow flavor of tarragon.

1 ruby red grapefruit, sectioned
1 head red leaf lettuce
1 avocado, peeled, pitted, and sliced
1/4 cup red onion, finely sliced

Arrange on a serving dish and drizzle with Tarragon Vinaigrette.

Tarragon Vinaigrette

2 tablespoons tarragon, finely chopped
2 teaspoons agave
1/4 cup lime juice

1/2 cup extra virgin olive oil
3 tablespoons Dijon mustard
1/4 cup white wine vinegar
black pepper

Shake well in a sealed container.

Greenmarket Salad | 1
MAKES 1-2 SERVINGS

Here we mix different aromas, textures, and colors to make a vibrant mixed salad with lots of variety. Great with a simple vinaigrette such as Apple Cider or Basic.

1 cup (handful) mixed greens
1 tablespoon fresh mint leaves, chopped
1 teaspoon fresh dill, chopped
4-5 cherry or grape tomatoes, quartered
1/4 English or seedless cucumber, sliced
2 tablespoons red onion, chopped
small handful sunflower sprouts
6-8 snow peas, sliced
1/2 ripe avocado, peeled, pitted, and sliced

Toss the mixed greens and herbs in a mixing bowl. Arrange on serving plates; top with the tomatoes, cucumber, red onion, sunflower sprouts, and snap peas. Arrange the avocado on top and drizzle with vinaigrette.

Mediterranean Salad | 1
MAKES 1-2 SERVINGS

Ideal with Raw Goddess Dressing (recipe page 169) but also delicious with any simple vinaigrette!

large handful (2 ounces) arugula
1/4 cup oil-packed sun-dried tomatoes, sliced
2 tablespoons black, pitted olives, rinsed and sliced
1/4 cup hearts of palm, sliced
1/2 cup cucumber, chopped
1/2 cup tomatoes, chopped
1 tablespoon capers

Mix all the ingredients together and drizzle with dressing.

Salsa Salad | 1
MAKES 2-4 SERVINGS

Fun fact: Raw corn digests as a vegetable, while cooked corn digests as a starch. So using raw corn in this salad makes it hearty and filling, but super easy and quick to digest. For an even heartier meal, don't skip the avocado!

1 ear fresh corn (1 cup)
8 cherry tomatoes, quartered
1/2 cup minced red onion (1/2 red onion)
2 medium cloves garlic, pressed or minced
1/2 cup diced red bell pepper
2 tablespoons pumpkin seeds, coarsely chopped
1/4 cup fresh cilantro, chopped
2 tablespoons extra virgin olive oil

2 tablespoons red wine vinegar

1 tablespoon fresh lemon juice

1/2 teaspoon sea salt

2 pinches ground cayenne

black pepper to taste

2 cups spinach, roughly torn

(Optional: 1 avocado, chopped)

Toss all the ingredients in a bowl and serve.

Sea Vegetable Salad with Ginger-Miso Dressing | 1
MAKES 2 SERVINGS

We wish more people understood the nutritious power of sea vegetables. Basic nori is most commonly found on the outside of sushi rolls, but hijiki and wakame shouldn't be overlooked! They are absolutely loaded with minerals and natural sources of protein and energy. And they are much more easily found than you'd think. Most health food stores have an array of different types of dried sea vegetables that simply get rehydrated in water.

1/4 cup dried wakame

1 cup warm water

1/2 cucumber, chopped

1/4 cup jicama, peeled and julienned

1 sheet nori, cut into strips

2 cups mixed greens

Soak the wakame in the warm water for 5–10 minutes, until tender. Drain. Place the mixed greens on a serving plate. Cover with the cucumber, jicama, and wakame. Top with nori strips and a drizzle of Ginger-Miso Dressing.

Ginger-Miso Dressing
MAKES 12 OUNCES

1/2 cup mellow white miso paste
1/3 cup agave nectar
1/3 cup apple cider vinegar
1/4 cup cold-pressed sesame oil
1/4 cup fresh lemon or lime juice
1/4 cup ginger, peeled and chopped.

Blend all the ingredients until smooth.

Shaved Fennel Salad | 1
MAKES 2 SERVINGS

This is a salad that is best when it's made with the right equipment. Yes, you can hand-slice the fennel very thinly, but it will take you some time and it's a little dangerous! A mandoline is a great purchase for thin-sliced veggies—just read the directions well and be careful!

1 medium fennel bulb, chop off top fronds and
    bottom 1/2 inch
1/2 lemon
2–3 tablespoons extra virgin olive oil
sea salt and ground black pepper to taste

Shave the fennel on a mandoline or slice thinly by hand. Toss with squeezed lemon juice and olive oil. Season with sea salt and pepper. This salad is best when dressed and tossed 15–30 minutes before serving.

Variation: Try adding chopped mint and thinly sliced avocado for a heartier salad.

Caesar Salad | 3
MAKES 1–2 SERVINGS

This garlicky lemon dressing tastes so much like the real thing, you'd never guess it was completely eggless and raw. Of course, adding the Parmesan (when two or more days out of a Cleanse) makes it that much more authentic. If using cheese, make sure it's imported and good quality—do not use anything that gets shaken out of that little green can!

¼ cup raw pine nuts
½ head romaine lettuce
¼ cup grated high-quality Parmesan Reggiano (when not
    cleansing)

Place the pine nuts in a dry pan. Over medium heat, toast the nuts until slightly brown, tossing gently while cooking. Remove from heat and set aside. Roughly chop the romaine and place in a bowl. Add ¼ cup Caesar dressing and toss until the lettuce is well coated. Place on serving plates and top with toasted pine nuts and Parmesan before serving.

Caesar Dressing
MAKES 6 OUNCES (ENOUGH FOR ABOUT 2 SERVINGS)

1 clove garlic, smashed with the flat side of a large knife
2 tablespoons Dijon mustard
2 tablespoons Macadamia Cream (see Dressings and Sauces)

2 teaspoons vegetarian Worcestershire sauce

2 teaspoons sea kelp flakes

2 tablespoons lemon juice (about 1 lemon)

2 tablespoons red wine vinegar

6 tablespoons extra virgin olive oil

In a small bowl, smash and whisk the garlic, mustard, and Macadamia Cream. Add the Worcestershire sauce, sea kelp flakes, lemon juice, and vinegar; continue to whisk. Drizzle in the olive oil and whisk well until the dressing is well emulsified (about 30–45 seconds). Serve.

Fresh Fava and Escarole Salad | 3
(can be a 1 without the Parmesan)
MAKES 1–2 SIDE SERVINGS

This salad is filling and delicious—a great way to enjoy escarole, which can be bitter when cooked but balances perfectly with the zesty lemon dressing. Don't be shy with the lemon here!

2 cups water

3/4 teaspoon sea salt + more to taste

1 cup shelled fava beans

1/4 head escarole, chopped into 1/2-inch strips

2 tablespoons fresh mint leaves, torn

1 1/2 teaspoons lemon juice (1/2 lemon)

1/2 teaspoon lemon zest, chopped (1 lemon)

1 tablespoon extra virgin olive oil

1 teaspoon apple cider vinegar

4–6 tablespoons Parmesan cheese (when not cleansing)

Place the water and ¹/4 teaspoon of the sea salt in a medium saucepan and bring to a boil. Have a bowl of ice water ready. Add the favas and allow the water to return to a boil. After about 60 seconds, prick the beans with a fork to check if tender. If ready, remove the beans from the water with a slotted spoon and immediately place in a bowl of ice water to blanch. Drain the beans and remove the outer peel. In a large bowl, combine the favas and the remaining ingredients. Toss until well combined and serve.

Lentil Salad | 3
MAKES 1-2 SERVINGS

This is a nontraditional salad in that there are very few actual "greens," but it's loaded with fresh veggie flavors and makes a great main dish. Travels well for picnics, too!

6 tablespoons dried green lentils (2 cups cooked)

1 ¹/4 cups water

¹/2 teaspoon salt

¹/2 cup roasted bell peppers, chopped

¹/4 cup finely minced onion

1 medium clove garlic, pressed

2 tablespoons chopped fresh basil

¹/4 cup coarsely chopped walnuts

1 tablespoon balsamic vinegar

2 teaspoons fresh lemon juice

2 teaspoons Bragg Liquid Aminos

2 tablespoons extra virgin olive oil

1 handful (1 cup) young dandelion leaves, chopped

black pepper to taste

Rinse the lentils. Combine the lentils, the water, and
¼ teaspoon of the salt in a medium saucepan; bring to a boil.
Reduce heat and cook at low temperature for about 15 minutes
or until the lentils are cooked and still a bit firm. Drain the
lentils and lightly rinse under cold water; allow to drain while
combining the remaining ingredients in a bowl. Add the lentils
and gently stir to combine. Serve.

Three Pea and Mint Salad with Shallot Vinaigrette | 3
(can be a 1 without the feta!)
MAKES 2-4 SIDE SERVINGS

*This fresh salad is ideal when eaten shortly after preparing, so
the greens stay bright green and crisp. Ideal for a warm spring or
summer day. Try to find organic "baby" peas as they are sweeter
than the larger ones. The feta adds a nice tangy touch, but you
can skip it if you're close to a Cleanse (or if you just don't like
it). Shallot Vinaigrette is ideal for this dish.*

1 cup sugar snap peas (8 ounces), strings removed

1/2 cup snow peas (4 ounces)

3 cups water

1/4 cup shelled frozen baby peas

2 tablespoons fresh mint, packed and roughly torn

Shallot Vinaigrette (see recipe on next page)

2-3 tablespoons organic feta cheese, crumbled (optional)

Bring 3 cups water to a boil in a saucepan. Have a bowl
of ice water ready. Place the sugar snap peas and snow peas
in the boiling water and allow to come back to boil. In about
60 seconds, quickly remove the peas with a slotted spoon and

place directly in the ice water to blanch. Drain the peas, rough chop, and place in a mixing bowl.

Bring the water back to a boil. Place the frozen baby peas in the water for 30 seconds. Quickly drain and rinse with cold water; add to the mixing bowl. Add mint and drizzle a small amount of vinaigrette. Toss well and add more vinaigrette as needed. Place on serving plates and top with feta.

Shallot Vinaigrette

$1/2$ shallot, finely minced

1 teaspoon Dijon mustard

1 tablespoon lemon juice

2 teaspoons white wine vinegar

$1 1/2$ tablespoons extra virgin olive oil

Place all the ingredients in a bowl and whisk well to combine.

Dressings and Sauces

Apple Cider Vinaigrette (ACV) | 1
MAKES 8 OUNCES

Unlike regular processed and pasteurized vinegar, ACV is alkaline, which helps balance the body's pH.

- 1/2 cup extra virgin olive oil
- 1/2 cup apple cider vinegar
- 1/4 teaspoon sea salt
- 1/4 cup agave nectar
- 1/2 teaspoon ground mustard seed
- 1 clove garlic

Blend all the ingredients until smooth.

Basic Vinaigrette | 1
MAKES ABOUT 1 CUP

This is a classic French recipe for vinaigrette that is perfect on any type of salad, really. You can play with the levels of vinegar for more or less acid, and try different types of vinegar to adjust the flavor.

3/4 cup extra virgin olive oil
1/4 cup red wine vinegar
3 tablespoons good-quality Dijon mustard

Place all the ingredients in a bowl and whisk well to combine.

Variations: Balsamic vinegar adds richness and sweetness, apple cider vinegar adds tartness, champagne vinegar has a delicate flavor, and red wine vinegar is great for a neutral balance.
Add chopped shallots, garlic, chives, basil, or tarragon for different aromas.

Easy Lemon-Tahini Dressing | 2
MAKES 4 OUNCES

Great on everything from simple greens to chopped veggie salads. This dressing is superversatile and an absolute favorite.

2 tablespoons fresh lemon juice
2 tablespoons sesame tahini
2 tablespoons mellow white miso
1 tablespoon water
1 teaspoon Nama Shoyu or Bragg Liquid Aminos

Place all the ingredients in a small container with a lid, and shake well until the ingredients are combined.

Macadamia Cream | 2
MAKES 4 OUNCES

This is a great base for creating many different salad dressings and spreads. You can experiment with your own creations by adding fresh chopped herbs or spices. Macadamias are rich in their own oils and therefore softer than other nuts, so they require less soaking time. If your blender isn't powerful enough to create a smooth result, you can push it through a fine strainer with a spatula.

- $1/2$ cup raw unsalted macadamia nuts, soaked 1–2 hours
- 2 teaspoons lemon juice
- $1/4$ teaspoon sea salt
- 6 tablespoons water
- 2 tablespoons extra virgin olive oil

Blend until very smooth and whipped. Store up to 5–6 days in the refrigerator until ready to use.

Pine Nut–Arugula Pesto | 2
MAKES 8 OUNCES

Another item that needs no raw translation. This makes a great topping for a simple summer tomato and onion salad, or as a spread for lettuce wraps or sprouted grain sandwiches on heartier days.

1 cup arugula, packed
1/4 cup fresh parsley, packed
1/4 cup fresh basil, packed
1/2 cup raw pine nuts
1/2 teaspoon sea salt
6 tablespoons extra virgin olive oil
black pepper

Place all the ingredients in a food processor. Process until chunky, scraping down the sides of the bowl frequently.

Ranch Dressing | 2
MAKES 10 OUNCES

This creamy and tangy dressing is a great replacement for the dairy-heavy original that has become a widely accepted way of smothering otherwise perfectly healthy salads across America. Don't get us started on this. The "dressing" has become the vehicle for the salad instead of a way to enhance its flavor! Use it as a dip for raw veggies, or drizzle it over a quartered head of iceberg and garnish with cherry tomatoes for a steakhouse-style wedge salad.

3/4 cup raw macadamia nuts, soaked 1 hour

1/4 cup fresh lemon juice

1 teaspoon sea salt

1/4 cup extra virgin olive oil

1/2 cup water

1 teaspoon dried parsley

1 teaspoon dried sage

1 1/2 tablespoons fresh chives, minced

Blend all the ingredients except the parsley, sage, and chives in a high-speed blender until smooth. Add the remaining ingredients and blend gently, just until the herbs and chives are broken down. Serve.

Raw Goddess Dressing | 2
MAKES 6 OUNCES (FOR 2-3 SALADS)

This dressing rivals any bottled goddess-style dressing, but is so much tastier when you make it fresh! The dried herbs give it a nice aroma, but if you have fresh chives on hand, finely chop 6–10 of them and throw them in for extra flavor. Ideal for soft lettuce mixes like Boston, red leaf, or mixed baby greens.

1/4 cup extra virgin olive oil

1/4 cup water

2 tablespoons organic sesame tahini

1 tablespoon apple cider vinegar

1 tablespoon Nama Shoyu

1 tablespoon lemon juice

1/4 teaspoon sea salt

1/2 small clove garlic

$^1/_4$ teaspoon dried parsley
$^1/_4$ teaspoon dried chives

Blend all the ingredients except the parsley, chives, and garlic until smooth.

Add the herbs and garlic and blend for only a few seconds until the remaining ingredients are broken down.

Main Dishes

Marinated Kale with Tahini Dressing |
MAKES 2 FIRST COURSE OR SIDE SERVINGS

The method isn't as complicated as it looks—the key is to really massage the kale with a little salt and whatever water is left on it after it's washed in order to break it down properly. If you omit this step, you'll wind up with tough and bitter kale. If you do it right, you're guaranteed to make this over and over. We've listed it as a main dish because it's very filling. Serve with a light soup or a sweet potato and you've got dinner.

1 bunch kale, rinsed and leaves torn from rib. Tear into smaller pieces.

$1/4$ cup unfiltered apple cider vinegar

$1/4$ cup fresh squeezed lemon juice (about 1 full lemon)

$1/4$ cup Nama Shoyu or $1/8$ cup Nama Shoyu plus $1/8$ cup Bragg Liquid Aminos *(We prefer it this way, but sometimes Bragg's is difficult to find in certain stores)*

2-3 tablespoons organic sesame tahini, depending on desired thickness

$1/2$ avocado and/or $1/2$ red bell pepper, both cut into bite-size strips or chunks

Celtic Sea Salt to taste
splash of agave nectar to taste

Pat dry the kale almost completely, place in a large bowl, and sprinkle a pinch or two of sea salt. Using your hands, massage the salt into the damp kale, squeezing well to thoroughly saturate the kale. (This massaging is what breaks down the kale and makes it soft enough to eat while raw.)

Place the vinegar, lemon juice, Nama Shoyu/Bragg's, garlic, and tahini into a small blender or food processer. *(We use the Magic Bullet, as seen on TV—haha!—but any small mixer will do.)* Pulse or blend until the mixture is well blended. The texture should be like a creamy salad dressing. If it's too thin, you can add a bit more tahini. If it's too tart for you, add a splash of agave nectar.

Pour the mixture over the massaged kale and work through well with your hands again. Let the salad marinate for at least 20–30 minutes. When ready to serve, add the avocado and/or pepper and mix through with a fork or spoon. The salad will keep in the refrigerator in a sealed container 2–3 days.

Roasted Portabella Mushroom | 1
MAKES 1-2 SERVINGS

For a complete meal of veggies and starch, the Creamy Rosemary Vinaigrette is also amazing on oven-roasted baby red potatoes.

2 large portabella mushrooms, rinsed and stems removed
1 tablespoon extra virgin olive oil
1/4 teaspoon sea salt
black pepper to taste
1/4 red bell pepper, sliced

2 tablespoons red onion, chopped
1 handful (1 cup) spinach

Preheat oven to 375°.

Slice the mushrooms in ½-inch pieces and place in a glass baking dish. Sprinkle olive oil, sea salt, and black pepper over the mushrooms and toss well. Bake 10–15 minutes until tender. On serving plates arrange the spinach, bell pepper, and red onions; top with mushrooms and drizzle with creamy Rosemary Vinaigrette.

Creamy Rosemary Vinaigrette | 2
MAKES 8 OUNCES (FOR 4 SALADS)

½ cup cashews, soaked 1 hour
¼ cup fresh rosemary, stems removed and chopped
¼ teaspoon sea salt
1 tablespoon lemon juice
6 tablespoons extra virgin olive oil
1 teaspoon white miso paste
2 tablespoons apple cider vinegar
¼ cup water
black pepper to taste

Blend until smooth.

Mango Lettuce Wrap | 2
MAKES 2 SERVINGS

Lettuce wraps are a great way to get lots of flavors and textures in one bite, while keeping it all self-contained. Play around with the ingredients. And don't miss out on the shrimp version when you're ready to add fish back into your plan!

8 romaine lettuce leaves

1/2 ripe mango, pitted and sliced

1/2 red bell pepper, seeded and sliced

1/2 ripe avocado, pitted, peeled, and sliced

1/4 cup alfalfa sprouts

sea salt to taste

1 tablespoon fresh mint, rough chopped

1 tablespoon fresh cilantro, rough chopped

1/4 cup raw or roasted cashews, chopped

8 long chives

(Can add grilled shrimp, 2 to 3 in each wrap.)

Remove the lighter green bottom of a romaine leaf where the stem becomes wider. Lay the leaf on your work space. Place 2 slices each of mango, bell pepper, and avocado lengthwise (along with stem) on the romaine leaf. (Optional: place one piece of grilled shrimp in each leaf.)

Top with a small amount of sprouts, a sprinkle of mint and cilantro, and a small pinch of sea salt. Roll the lettuce leaf tightly and tie with one chive. Continue with the remaining lettuce leaves. Serve with Sweet Lime Dipping Sauce.

Sweet Lime Dipping Sauce
MAKES 6 OUNCES

1/2 cup pitted dates, soaked 15 minutes
1/2 cup fresh lime juice (1 1/2 limes)
4 teaspoons agave nectar
1/2 teaspoon sea salt
2 tablespoons water
pinch ground cayenne pepper

Blend until smooth.

Roasted Fennel, Beets, and Sweet Potatoes | 2
MAKES 1–2 SERVINGS

Simple roasted root vegetables should not be overlooked as just a vegetarian's lack of creativity! These are packed with nutrients and absolutely delicious, especially when something warm and wintry is in order.

1/2 fennel bulb, green stems removed, halved, and cut into
    1/4-inch slices
1 medium red beet, peeled, halved, and cut into 1/4-inch slices
1/2 medium sweet potato (7 1/2 ounces)
2 tablespoons extra virgin olive oil
1/2 teaspoon sea salt
black pepper to taste
1 tablespoon rosemary, stems removed and finely chopped
1 tablespoon thyme, stems removed and finely chopped

Preheat oven to 400°.

Toss all the ingredients in a glass baking dish. Spread the vegetables into a single layer and bake in the center of the oven for 30–35 minutes until the beets can easily be pierced by a fork. Serve warm.

Spaghetti Squash | 2
SERVES 2 AS AN ENTRÉE PORTION

Spaghetti squash is pretty much the coolest-looking vegetable ever. This is a satisfying and filling substitute for starchy, dense noodles when you're really having a craving for some Italian comfort food. You can even top it with organic pasta sauce for the whole nine yards.

1 medium spaghetti squash
3 tablespoons extra virgin olive oil
salt and pepper to taste
1/4 cup grated Parmesan (optional)

Preheat oven to 400°.

Poke the spaghetti squash with a fork on all sides to prevent bursting in the oven. Roast for 1 hour. Remove from oven and cut in half. (Be careful! *Hot!*) Scoop out all the seeds with a spoon and discard. Using a fork and holding the squash in place with an oven mitt, gently scrape down away the insides of the squash, which will unfold in long spaghetti-like strands.

Heat the olive oil in a large saucepan and add the squash, salt, and pepper. Mix well and heat over medium flame for 3 minutes. Finish with Parmesan and/or tomato sauce if desired.

Asian Cold Noodles with
Spicy Almond Dressing | 3
MAKES 1-2 SERVINGS

Reminiscent of every Chinese restaurant's classic cold noodles with peanut sauce appetizer, only this one gives you energy instead of inducing a food coma!

4 ounces buckwheat soba noodles
1/2 cup cucumber, peeled, seeded, and chopped
1/4 cup scallions, sliced
1/2 red bell pepper, seeded and sliced
1/2 cup mung bean sprouts
1/2 cup Spicy Almond Dressing
1/2 lime for garnish

Bring a saucepan of water to a boil and add the noodles. Lower heat and cook at a low simmer for 6–8 minutes until the soba is tender. Remove from heat. Put the noodles in a strainer and rinse with cool water. Drain. Place the noodles in a bowl and add the cucumber, scallions, and red bell pepper. Toss with Spicy Almond Dressing. Top with bean sprouts and a squeeze of lime before serving.

Spicy Almond Dressing
MAKES 8 OUNCES

1/2 cup raw or roasted almond butter
6 tablespoons tomatoes, chopped
2 tablespoons Nama Shoyu *or* Bragg Liquid Aminos
2 tablespoons extra virgin olive oil

3 teaspoons fresh lime juice

2 teaspoons agave nectar

3/4 teaspoon ginger, peeled and chopped

1/4–1/2 teaspoon ground cayenne pepper

1/2 teaspoon sea salt

Blend all the ingredients in a high-speed blender until completely smooth.

Brown Rice Sushi Rolls | 3

Labor intensive, maybe—but nothing impresses guests like perfect hand-rolled sushi, and once you get the hang of it, it's quite easy!

1 1/4 cups water

sea salt to taste

1/2 cup brown rice

2 tablespoons brown rice vinegar

1 tablespoon agave nectar

Bring the water to a boil and add a pinch of sea salt. Stir in the rice and reduce heat to low—cover and let simmer for 25 minutes. Remove from heat and let sit covered for 5 minutes. With a fork, toss the rice with the vinegar, agave, and salt (to taste).

1/4 cup Nama Shoyu

2 tablespoons sesame oil

1 large portabella mushroom, sliced into 1/2-inch strips

1/2 avocado, pitted, peeled, and sliced

1/2 English cucumber, seeded, peeled, and sliced lengthwise
    into 1/2-inch strips

pickled radish, rinsed and sliced lengthwise (available at Asian
    specialty stores)
small handful sunflower sprouts
2 sheets untoasted nori
1 teaspoon wasabi
pickled ginger for garnish
Nama Shoyu for dipping

Place the Shoyu and oil in a shallow bowl and whisk with a
fork until emulsified; add the mushroom, toss well, and let sit
5–10 minutes. Gently squeeze the mushroom slices dry and place
on your work space with the avocado, cucumber, pickled radish,
and sunflower sprouts. Place a bamboo rolling mat on the work
space and top with 1 nori sheet, shiny side down. Spread the
brown rice in a thin layer on $3/4$ of the nori closest to you.

Across the center of the rice, place a few slices each of
mushrooms, avocado, cucumber, radish, and sprouts. Tightly
roll the sushi by starting with the edge closest to you, and pulling
forward as you roll. (This may take practice!) Slice each roll into 6
pieces. Serve with wasabi, pickled ginger, and extra Nama Shoyu.

Napoleon with Goat Cheese | 3
MAKES 1-2 SERVINGS

*This dish makes an elegant presentation when all the colors
and textures are layered on top of each other. A beautiful main
course for a dinner party.*

2 portabella mushrooms, stemmed and sliced into $1/2$-inch
    pieces
1 tablespoon extra virgin olive oil
$1/4$ teaspoon sea salt
black pepper to taste

1 clove garlic, pressed

1 teaspoon fresh thyme, finely chopped

3–4 large basil leaves

1 large red tomato, sliced into 1/4-inch pieces

4 ounces organic goat cheese, sliced into 1/4-inch pieces

extra olive oil for garnish

Preheat oven to 375°.

Toss the mushroom slices with the olive oil, salt, pepper, garlic, and thyme. Place the mushrooms in a small pan in a single layer. Bake 10–12 minutes until tender. Place 3 mushroom slices, side by side, on each serving dish. Top with a basil leaf, a slice of tomato, a slice of goat cheese, and another basil leaf. Garnish with a drizzle of olive oil and a pinch of black pepper before serving.

Oven-Roasted Tilapia | 3
MAKES 2 SERVINGS

This method works well with any firm-fleshed fish, but tilapia is our favorite. The oven packet method is also ideal for small kitchens, when you don't want the whole house stinking of fish! And cleanup is ridiculously simple. Serve with a salad and some marinated kale for a complete meal.

2 tilapia filets

2 tablespoons extra virgin olive oil

1/2 lemon, remaining half cut into quarters for serving

salt and pepper to taste

2 tablespoons Old Bay (a salt-free Cajun seasoning) or chili powder

2 sheets of aluminum foil, enough to wrap each filet separately and close tightly

Preheat oven to 350°.

Lay a foil sheet on the counter, add a little olive oil, and place one filet in the center. Sprinkle the filet on both sides with half the seasoning, salt and pepper, and a quarter of the lemon. Finish the top with a bit more olive oil.

Seal the packet closed by folding the middle over and then folding in the ends. You want it to be sealed but not airtight. Repeat with the other filet and ingredients. Roast on the center rack for 20 minutes. Serve with the remaining lemon wedges.

Spicy Tuna Tartare | 3
MAKES 2 APPETIZER SERVINGS

The secret to the elegant presentation of this dish is a simple plastic ring mold. You can find them in any kitchen specialty section and they make all the difference! Note: This recipe is spectacular when it starts with a layer of simple guacamole in the ring mold, and then layers the tuna combination on top, but it's a no-no for food combining rules. Still, if you want to live a little...

8 ounces sushi grade tuna, diced into 1/4-inch cubes (once you trim and cut down, you'll have about 6 ounces)

1 teaspoon sesame oil

2 teaspoons Nama Shoyu

1 teaspoon lime juice

1 teaspoon chili sauce

1/2 teaspoon toasted sesame seeds (optional, for garnish)

Combine all the ingredients in a bowl and let stand for 10 minutes before serving. Can be served with rice crackers or tortilla chips for a nicer presentation (though a food combining no-no).

Guacamole

¹/₂ avocado
1 teaspoon lime juice
pinch sea salt

Mash all the ingredients together and serve on top of Tuna Tartare pressed into a ring mold.

Steamed Vegetables with Green Curry Sauce | 3
MAKES 1-2 SERVINGS

This Thai-inspired dish has an exotic flavor and a real kick of heat from the Green Curry Sauce.

¹/₂ cup quinoa
³/₄ cup cold water
¹/₂ teaspoon sea salt
¹/₂ bunch asparagus, hard, woody ends snapped off
¹/₂ red bell pepper, stem removed, seeded and sliced
¹/₂ medium zucchini, sliced into ¹/₂-inch pieces

To prepare quinoa:
Soak for 15–30 minutes. Drain and rinse through a sieve until the water runs through clean. Place in a pot with ³/₄ cup water and ¹/₄ teaspoon sea salt. Bring to a simmer, cover, and cook 20 minutes. Remove from heat and let sit covered for 5 minutes. Fluff the quinoa with a fork and set aside.

To steam vegetables:
Pour 1 inch of water in a saucepan. Place the vegetables in a steamer and position over the water. Sprinkle the remaining sea salt over the vegetables; bring the water to a boil, cover, lower

heat, and let steam for 15 minutes until tender. Place the quinoa in the center of serving dishes and top with steamed vegetables. Drizzle Green Curry Sauce over the vegetables and serve.

Green Curry Sauce
MAKES 12 OUNCES

3/4 cup raw cashews, soaked 1–2 hours

4 teaspoons fresh lime juice

1 1/2 tablespoons jalapeño chilies, seeded and minced

1/4 cup chopped scallions

1 tablespoon fresh ginger, peeled and chopped

2 tablespoons fresh lemongrass, chopped

2 tablespoons fresh basil

1 teaspoon curry powder

1/4 teaspoon sea salt

1 1/2 teaspoon raw agave nectar

3/4 cup water

Blend all the ingredients in a high-speed blender until smooth.

Veggie Tacos | 3
(2 without cheese)
MAKES 2 SERVINGS

Sprouted corn tortillas are usually in the freezer section of a good health food store. Their chewy texture and nutty flavor are absolutely amazing! This is a great dinner for a group, where everyone can dress up their tacos according to their own taste. Start with Gazpacho and you've got yourself a fiesta!

2 sprouted corn tortillas (sprouted grain tortillas will work, too,
   if sprouted corn is hard to find)
Guacamole (choose from Yankee or Cowboy recipes)
Pico de Gallo (see below)
1/2 cup raw, organic cheese of your choice, crumbled
1/2 cup romaine lettuce, shredded

Drizzle a bit of olive oil in a frying pan over low heat. Place one tortilla at a time in the pan; heat on each side just until warm. In the center of each tortilla, place a dollop of Guacamole (see recipe page 195) and an equal amount of Pico de Gallo. Top with the desired amount of cheese and romaine lettuce. Fold the sides of the burrito in and roll tightly before serving.

Pico de Gallo

4 Roma tomatoes, seeded and minced
1/2 cup red onion, minced
2 tablespoons lime juice (from 1/2 lime)
1/2 teaspoon salt
black pepper to taste
2 tablespoons fresh cilantro, well chopped

Mix all the ingredients in a bowl.

Small Dishes and Sides

Celery Root Remoulade | 2
MAKES 2-4 SERVINGS

Celery root (or celeriac) is the knobby, homely cousin of the more regal celery, but looks aren't everything—its flavor is ten times as delicious. This is a traditional French salad that we've translated into raw and we think it's actually way better than the mayonnaise-y original.

1 medium celery root, peeled and cut into matchsticks or grated

1/2 cup Macadamia Cream (see Dressings and Sauces)

2 tablespoons Dijon mustard

4 teaspoons white wine vinegar

1/2 teaspoon sea salt

black pepper to taste

2 teaspoons celery seed

1 teaspoon extra virgin olive oil

2 teaspoons fresh parsley, rough chopped

Place the celery root in a medium-sized bowl and set aside. In a small bowl, whisk together the Macadamia Cream, mustard, vinegar, salt, pepper, celery seed, and oil. Add the mixture to the celery root—just enough to coat it. Gently fold in the parsley and serve.

Raw Fennel and Cabbage Slaw | 2
MAKES 2-4 SERVINGS

This crunchy creamy slaw travels well for picnics. The celery seed is the magic ingredient, believed to help lower blood pressure, reduce inflammation, aid in digestion, and lower cholesterol— don't skip it!

$1/8$ red cabbage, sliced into fine strips with a mandoline
$1/2$ large fennel bulb, sliced into fine strips with a mandoline
$3/4$ cup Pine Nut Mayo
1 tablespoon celery seed

Toss all the ingredients together and refrigerate until ready to serve.

Pine Nut Mayo
MAKES 10 OUNCES

$3/4$ cup raw pine nuts, soaked 30 minutes
$1/4$ cup apple cider vinegar
2 tablespoons agave nectar
2 tablespoons water
$1/4$ teaspoon ground mustard seed
1 teaspoon sea salt
black pepper to taste
2 tablespoons extra virgin olive oil

Blend all ingredients until smooth.

Steamed Artichoke | 2
MAKES 1-2 SERVINGS

We think most people really believe that artichokes are born in glass jars with oily seasonings. They have no idea what they are missing. Beginners: Don't let the natural packaging of this amazing vegetable scare you—just work your way from the outside in by pulling off the leaves and dipping them in the Lemon Aioli, then scrape the meat from the bottom of the leaf with your teeth. When you get to the leaves that aren't meaty, you can discard them and scrape out the bottom of the choke to reveal the delicious and nutrient-packed heart. Cut into chunks and dip away! Serve warm or chilled.

1 large artichoke
2 slices fresh lemon
pinch sea salt

Rinse the artichoke and remove the lower petals. Cut the stem off close to the base. In a deep saucepan, add 1 inch water. Add the lemon slices and salt to the water. Place a steam rack or steamer basket over the water and place the artichoke on the rack, base down. Cover and bring to a boil. Lower heat and then steam for 30–45 minutes, until a petal near the center can easily be pulled out. Serve with Lemon Aioli and a *big* side bowl for discarded leaves.

Lemon Aioli

1/2 cup raw cashews, soaked 1 hour
1/4 cup water
3 tablespoons fresh lemon juice

3–4 garlic cloves

$1/4$ teaspoon ground mustard seeds

pinch sea salt

black pepper to taste

$1/2$ cup extra virgin olive oil

Blend all the ingredients in a high-speed blender until smooth and well emulsified.

Sweet Potato Mash | 2
MAKES 1–2 SERVINGS

Shhh: If you want this fragrant and colorful dish to taste really *indulgent, add a tablespoon of good-quality organic low- or no-salt butter when mashing!*

1 medium-sized sweet potato or yam, peeled and sliced into
    $1/2$-inch pieces

$1/4$ teaspoon sea salt

black pepper to taste

2 teaspoons extra virgin olive oil

2 tablespoons fresh orange juice

$1/4$ teaspoon garam masala (an Indian seasoning available in
    most food stores)

Preheat oven to 400°.

Toss the potatoes in a glass baking dish with sea salt and pepper. Bake for 25 minutes. Place the potatoes in a bowl with the remaining ingredients. Mash with a fork until smooth and serve warm.

Snacks

Guacamole Two Ways | 1
MAKES 1 SERVING EACH (4 OUNCES)

We go back and forth over which recipe we prefer, as the subtle changes really make a big difference. Cowboy is piquant, chunky, and very flavorful while Yankee is simpler and probably better if you plan to spend some up-close-and-personal time where dragon breath is not an option.

Yankee

¹/₂ avocado, peeled
1 teaspoon lemon juice (adjust to taste)
¹/₄ teaspoon sea salt (adjust to taste)
1–2 pinches cayenne pepper

Cowboy

¹/₂ avocado, peeled
1 teaspoon lime juice (adjust to taste)
¹/₄ teaspoon sea salt (adjust to taste)
1 teaspoon red onion, finely minced

¹/₄ clove garlic, minced (¹/₂ teaspoon)
¹/₄–¹/₂ teaspoon jalapeño, minced
1 tablespoon tomato, seeded and minced
¹/₂ teaspoon cilantro, chopped

Sesame Dip | 2
MAKES 8 OUNCES

6 tablespoons almond butter
5 tablespoons sesame tahini
2 tablespoons extra virgin olive oil
5 tablespoons Bragg Liquid Aminos
2 tablespoons apple cider vinegar
1 clove garlic, pressed
pinch cayenne pepper

Whisk all the ingredients together, or blend in a food processor for a smoother consistency.

Spicy Edamame Hummus | 2
MAKES 10 OUNCES

Edamame makes an absolutely delicious replacement for tough-to-digest chickpeas. This stuff will blow your mind, no joke. Great as a spread on lettuce wraps or an hors d'oeuvre dipper with cut red peppers, carrot, and celery sticks.

3 ¹/₄ cups water
1 ¹/₂ teaspoons sea salt
1 cup frozen, shelled edamame (8 ounces)
¹/₄ cup sesame tahini
3 tablespoons extra virgin olive oil

3 tablespoons fresh lemon juice
1 clove garlic
1/2 teaspoon chili powder
pinch cayenne

In a saucepan, place 3 cups of water and 1 teaspoon of the salt; bring to a boil. Add the edamame and allow the water to come back to a boil. Cook, uncovered, for 5 minutes. Drain the edamame and place in a high-speed blender or food processor with the remaining ingredients. Blend until smooth and serve.

Sweet Potato and Beetroot Crisps | 2
MAKES 1–2 SERVINGS

Colorful and yummy, these crisps are way better than anything you could find in a bag.

1 medium sweet potato or yam, peeled
1 medium red beet, peeled
4 teaspoons extra virgin olive oil plus a little extra
sea salt and black pepper to taste

Preheat oven to 400°.

Slice the potatoes very thinly using a mandoline; place in a bowl. Slice the beet thinly with the mandoline and place in a separate bowl. Add 2 teaspoons olive oil to each bowl, along with salt and black pepper. Toss the ingredients well. Oil 2 cookie sheets with extra olive oil; on one, spread the potato slices in a single layer, and do the same with the beet slices on the other. If desired, sprinkle a bit more salt and pepper. Bake the sweet potatoes for 20 minutes and the beets for 25 minutes. Halfway through, flip slices. Remove from the oven and allow to cool completely before serving.

Brunch

Even though all good recipe collections include amazing breakfast items, we're calling this section "Brunch," since if you've been reading carefully, you already know that in our world, breakfast means juice or, at most, fresh fruit.

So while we don't want to confuse things or lead you astray, we also want you to have options at the ready on days when there's just no substitute. But try to do your body a favor and at least wait 'til you've been up and at 'em for a couple of hours.

Classic Veggie Omelettes | 3
MAKES 1 OMELETTE

We love eggs as much as the next girl. Here is a basic omelette recipe followed by suggested tried-and-true ingredients for great-tasting flavor combinations. A perfectly folded omelette takes practice, so keep at it!

3 organic eggs
1 teaspoon organic unsalted butter or cold-pressed olive oil
salt and fresh-cracked pepper to taste
1/3 cup total additional ingredients (next page)

Crack the eggs into a small nonreactive bowl and beat well with a fork. Add the salt and pepper. Heat a small sauté pan over medium heat and add the butter or oil. When the pan is hot (test it by flicking a drop of water and make sure it dances!), pour in the eggs. Using a rubber spatula, loosen the edges away from the sides of the pan as they cook, picking up the pan to swirl the runnier parts closer to the edges of the pan. When the center starts to set, add the additional ingredients and scatter them throughout the eggs.

Use the rubber spatula to fold half of the omelette over and continue cooking until the middle sets completely. Flip over to finish cooking the other side. Total cooking time should be about 7 minutes. You may need to lower the heat during the process to prevent burning.

Additional Ingredients

Sautéed spinach and goat cheese (sauté spinach ahead until wilted)

Sautéed mushrooms, caramelized onions, and Gruyère (sauté mushrooms and/or onions ahead of time in olive oil until soft and browned)

Roasted red peppers, asparagus, and goat cheese

Sprouted Bagel with Tangy Dill Spread | 3
MAKES 1-2 SERVINGS

A shmear of this Tangy Dill Spread replaces cream cheese and makes every day taste like Sunday, dahling! Add some cured salmon (gravlax) when not cleansing!

1 sprouted grain bagel
Tangy Dill Spread
1/4 cucumber, sliced
1/4 red onion, sliced
1 tablespoon capers
black pepper to taste

Slice the bagel in half lengthwise and toast. Spread Tangy Dill Spread over each half. On the bottom half, top the Spread with red onion slices, cucumber, capers, and black pepper to taste. Top with the other half of the bagel and serve!

Tangy Dill Spread
MAKES 10 OUNCES

1 cup raw cashews, soaked 1 hour
1/4 cup fresh lemon juice
3/4 teaspoon sea salt
1/4 cup water
1/4 cup extra virgin olive oil
1 tablespoon fresh dill, chopped

Place all the ingredients except the dill in a high-speed blender or food processor and blend until smooth. Add the dill and pulse chop just until the dill is broken down.

CEREALS

Sprouted grain cereals are definitely the closest we'd recommend you go to a store-bought breakfast, and even then, it should be at least two days away from your Cleanse on either end. A great homemade cereal that's easy to digest and completely gluten-free can be made from preparing quinoa according to the regular cooking directions, and then adding a dash of cinnamon and a touch of raw honey, agave, or real maple syrup. Resist the urge to sprinkle dried or fresh fruit here—you're in for a world of pain (read: gas) if you opt to do that!

The best breakfast truly consists of fresh fruit. Fresh-cut papaya, watermelon, or pineapple (alone, not mixed, please!) are some of the best ways to start your day. Which brings us to juices and smoothies. There are limitless options when it comes to juice combinations, but here are our favorites, which are sure to become yours.

Juices and Nut Milks

The following recipes make one 16-ounce drink. Remember the daily juices for each level:

Renovation: three fruit juices, two green juices, and one nut milk

Foundation: two fruit juices, three green juices, and one nut milk

Excavation: one fruit juice, four green juices, and one nut milk

FRUIT JUICES

Apple-Pear-Beet-Ginger

1 1/2 Granny Smith apple
1 1/2 D'Anjou/Bosc pear
3 small or 1 large (3 1/8 ounces) red beet
1-inch piece ginger

Wash the all ingredients. Quarter and core the apples and pears. Cut the beets into pieces that will fit through a juicer. Run all the ingredients through the juicer. Run any wet pulp back through the juicer. Scrape off the foam and serve.

Blackberry-Peach

1 cup frozen blackberries
1 cup frozen peaches
1 1/2 cups liquid (rice milk)

Combine all ingredients and blend until smooth.

Blueberry-Apple-Vanilla

1 cup fresh blueberries
$1/2$ Granny Smith apple, chopped
1 fresh banana
$1/2$ teaspoon vanilla extract
1 $1/2$ cups ice

Combine all ingredients and blend until smooth.

Blueberry-Pineapple

1 cup frozen blueberries
1 cup frozen pineapple
1 $1/2$ cups liquid (rice milk)

Combine all ingredients and blend until smooth.

Carrot-Apple-Ginger

3 medium carrots
2 Granny Smith apples
1- to 2-inch piece ginger (according to taste)

Wash all the ingredients. Cut the apples into quarters and remove the cores. Run all the ingredients through the juicer. Run any wet pulp back through the juicer. Scrape off the foam and serve.

Carrot-Apple-Parsley-Beet-Orange

2 medium carrots
1 1/2 Granny Smith apple
1 medium red beet
1 navel orange
small handful (1/2 ounce) parsley

Wash the carrots, apple, beet, and parsley. Core and quarter the apple, and cut the beet into pieces that will fit through a juicer. Cut the peel away from the orange. Remove any long stems from the parsley. Run all the ingredients through the juicer. Run any wet pulp back through the juicer. Scrape off the foam and serve.

Cherry-Banana-Peach

1 cup frozen cherries
1 frozen banana
1 cup frozen peaches
2 cups liquid (rice milk)

Combine all ingredients and blend until smooth.

Cran-Banana

1 cup frozen cranberries
1 frozen banana
1 1/2 cups liquid (rice milk)

Combine all ingredients and blend until smooth.

Frozen Cherry-Lime

1 1/2 cup frozen cherries
1/4 cup lime juice (from 2 limes)
1 fresh banana
3/4 cup ice

Combine all ingredients and blend until smooth.

Grape-Cucumber-Pear (very clean-tasting)

1 pint (10 ounces) green grapes
1/2 large cucumber
1 D'Anjou/Bosc pear
1-inch piece of ginger

Wash all the ingredients. Cut the cucumber into pieces that will fit through a juicer; quarter and core the pear. Run all the ingredients through the juicer. Run any wet pulp back through the juicer. Scrape off foam and serve.

Grapefruit-Strawberry-Mint

1/2 grapefruit
1 pint (10 ounces) strawberries
small handful mint

Cut the peel away from the grapefruit. Wash the strawberries and mint. Cut the stems from the strawberries; remove any hard, woody stems from the mint. Run all the ingredients

through the juicer. Run any wet pulp back through the juicer.
Scrape off the foam and serve.

Mango-Red Cherry

1 cup frozen mango
1 cup frozen cherries
1 1/2 cups liquid (rice milk)

Combine all ingredients and blend until smooth.

Mango-Strawberry

1 fresh, ripe mango, peeled and chopped
1 cup fresh strawberries, stemmed
1 1/2 cups ice

Combine all ingredients and blend until smooth.

Mango-Strawberry

1 cup frozen mango
1 cup frozen strawberry
1 1/2 cups liquid (rice milk)

Combine all ingredients and blend until smooth.

Mixed Berry-Banana

1/2 cup fresh strawberries, chopped
1/2 cup fresh raspberries
1/2 cup fresh blueberries
1 fresh banana
1 1/2 cups ice

Combine all ingredients and blend until smooth.

Mixed Berry-Kale

1 cup frozen mixed berries
1 frozen banana
3 medium stalks fresh kale, stems removed
1 1/2 cups liquid (rice milk)

Combine all ingredients and blend until smooth.

Orange-Pomegranate

2 Valencia oranges
2 pomegranates

Cut the oranges and pomegranates in half. Juice the halves with an electric or hand citrus juicer. Serve.

Pear-Banana-Blueberry

1 fresh, ripe pear
1 fresh banana
3/4 cup fresh blueberries
1 1/2 cup ice

Combine all ingredients and blend until smooth.

Pineapple-Beet-Ginger-Pear

1/4 pineapple
1 medium beet
1 D'Anjou/Bosc pear
1-inch piece ginger

Cut the skin from the pineapple and slice it into pieces that will fit through a juicer. Wash the beet, pear, and ginger. Cut the beet into pieces that will fit through a juicer. Quarter and core the pear. Run all the ingredients through the juicer. Run any wet pulp back through the juicer. Scrape off the foam and serve.

Pineapple-Mango

1/2 cup frozen pineapple
1/2 cup frozen mango
1 cup liquid (rice milk)

Combine all ingredients and blend until smooth.

Pineapple-Mango-Banana-Strawberry
MAKES 20 OUNCES

$1/2$ cup frozen pineapple
$1/2$ cup frozen mango
$1/2$ frozen banana
$1/2$ cup frozen strawberry
$1 1/2$ cups liquid (rice milk)

Combine all ingredients and blend until smooth.

Pineapple-Mint

2 cups fresh pineapple, chopped
10–15 leaves fresh mint (according to taste)
$1 1/2$ cups ice

Combine all ingredients and blend until smooth.

Pineapple-Orange-Celery

$1/4$ pineapple
$1 1/2$ navel oranges
3 stalks celery
small handful ($1/8$ ounce or 1–2 sprigs) mint

Cut the skin from the pineapple and slice it into pieces that will fit through a juicer. Cut the peel from the orange. Wash the celery and mint. Remove any thick, woody stems from the mint and remove any leaves from the celery. Run all the ingredients through the juicer. Run any wet pulp back through the juicer. Scrape off the foam and serve.

Pineapple-Pear-Lemongrass

1/8 pineapple
1 1/2 D'Anjou/Bosc pear
4-inch piece (3/4 ounce) fresh lemongrass

Cut the skin from the pineapple and slice it into pieces that will fit through a juicer. Wash, quarter, and core the pears. Peel away any dry outer layers of lemongrass. Run all the ingredients through the juicer. Run any wet pulp back through the juicer. Scrape off the foam and serve.

Pineapple-Raspberry-Mint

1 cup frozen pineapple
1 cup frozen raspberries
small handful fresh mint
1 1/2 cups liquid (rice milk)

Combine all ingredients and blend until smooth.

Raspberry-Banana-Orange

1 cup fresh raspberry
1 fresh banana
1 orange, peeled
1 cup ice

Combine all ingredients and blend until smooth.

Strawberry-Apple-Beet

1 pint (10 ounces) fresh strawberries
1 medium Granny Smith apple
1 medium red beet
1-inch piece ($3/4$ ounces) ginger

Wash all the ingredients. Cut the stems from the strawberries. Cut the apple into quarters and remove the core. Cut the beet into pieces that will fit through a juicer. Run all the ingredients through the juicer. Run any wet pulp back through the juicer. Scrape off the foam and serve.

Strawberry-Banana

1 cup frozen strawberries
1 frozen banana
1 1/2 cups liquid (rice milk)

Combine all ingredients and blend until smooth.

Strawberry-Kiwi

1 cup fresh strawberries, chopped
2 fresh, ripe (slightly soft) kiwis, peeled
1 1/2 cups ice

Combine all ingredients and blend until smooth.

Vanilla-Banana-Cinnamon

2 fresh bananas
1 teaspoon ground cinnamon
Seeds from $1/4$ fresh vanilla bean
$1/2$ teaspoon vanilla extract
pinch sea salt
1 $1/2$ cups ice

Combine all ingredients and blend until smooth.

Watermelon! (lime or mint optional)

$1/8$ fresh watermelon (about 16 ounces), chopped

Blend until smooth.

GREEN JUICES

Greens with Apple

handful (3 ounces) spinach
3 medium stalks (3 ounces) kale
2 Golden Delicious apples
$1/2$ large cucumber
small handful ($1/2$ ounce) parsley, long stems removed
1 lemon

Wash all the ingredients. Cut the peel from the lemon.
Quarter and core the apples; cut the cucumber into pieces that
will fit through a juicer. Run all the ingredients through the

juicer. Run any wet pulp back through the juicer. Scrape off the foam and serve. For Apple/Ginger variation, add 1-inch piece of peeled ginger when juicing.

Spinach-Blueberry-Apple-Lemon

small handful (1–2 ounces) spinach
1 pint (10 ounces) blueberries
1 Granny Smith apple
1 lemon

Wash spinach, blueberries, and apple. Core the apple and cut it into quarters. Cut the peel away from the lemon. Run all the ingredients through the juicer. Run any wet pulp back through the juicer. Scrape off the foam and serve.

Spinach-Carrot-Pineapple-Cilantro

handful (3 ounces) spinach
2 medium carrots
1/4 pineapple
small bunch (1/2 ounce) cilantro (optional)
1 lime
1 drop liquid cayenne

Wash the spinach, carrots, and cilantro (optional). Cut the peel away from the pineapple and cut it into pieces that will fit through juicer. Cut the peel away from the lime. Run spinach, carrots, pineapple, cilantro (optional), and lime through the juicer. Run any wet pulp back through juicer. Scrape off the foam, stir in liquid cayenne, and serve.

NUT MILKS

Easy Cashew Milk

1/2 cup raw cashews, soaked 1 hour (in 1 cup water)
2 cups filtered water
1 1/2 teaspoon extra virgin coconut oil
1/4 teaspoon vanilla extract
2 teaspoons agave
pinch sea salt

Drain the nuts. Combine all the ingredients and blend until completely smooth. Store in a refrigerator for up to 5 days. Shake well before use.

Raw Chocolate Milk

1/2 cup raw cashews, soaked 1 hour
2 cups filtered water
3 tablespoons raw cacao nibs
1 teaspoon vanilla extract
2 1/2 tablespoons agave nectar
2 teaspoons extra virgin coconut oil
pinch sea salt

Drain the nuts. Combine all the ingredients and blend until completely smooth. Store in a refrigerator for up to 5 days. Shake well before use.

Index